Praise for
Why Woo-Woo Works

'We sometimes call things "woo-woo" not because we're experts on those subjects, but because we're not experts and we haven't dived into all the available science and research. In this book, David has done a stellar job in gathering the science and philosophy behind a range of seemingly woo-woo subjects and shown that they are, in fact, "true-woo."'

VEX KING, #1 SUNDAY TIMES BEST-SELLING AUTHOR OF GOOD VIBES, GOOD LIFE

'Dr. David Hamilton is one of the leading experts in the field of the mind-body connection. As a scientist, he bridges real science with human potential in order to prove to you how powerful you really are. This book will change your mind.'

DR. JOE DISPENZA, NEW YORK TIMES BEST-SELLING AUTHOR OF YOU ARE THE PLACEBO

'Science has historically looked askance when faced with traditional healing systems. We now realize that alternative therapies and Western methods can be used together to reach a state of lasting wellness.'

DEEPAK CHOPRA

'Why Woo-Woo Works is one of the clearest and most accurate expositions of alternative mind-body practices that I've had the pleasure to read. Hamilton also offers explanations that help to demystify the woo-woo taboo. A delightful and inspiring read.'

DEAN RADIN, PH.D., CHIEF SCIENTIST, INSTITUTE OF NOETIC SCIENCES

'David is an incredibly inspirational man who I'm proud to call a friend. His work has changed the lives of many and he stands out because he always strives to explore and answer the difficult questions using evidence and science, which in a world full of misinformation, is needed. A truly wonderful and fascinating book. A must-read!'

DR. PUNAM KRISHAN, GP, WRITER, AND BROADCASTER

'David's emotionally moving and scientifically enlightening book delves deep into the big questions of spirituality and science. Read this book to open your mind and heart to the tremendous power of alternative therapies.'
DR. NILESH SATGURU, GP AND HIGH-PERFORMANCE COACH

'Reading this book is like David giving us a scientific toy arm to finally be able to scratch that itch on our back in that unreachable spot for those of us who have resonated with woo-woo since day one, but haven't had the evidence-based research compiled all in one place to back up what we feel and have experienced to be true. If medical students and sceptics everywhere were required to read this book, the world would be a more harmonious and healthy place.'
KELLY NOONAN GORES, DIRECTOR AND EXECUTIVE PRODUCER OF THE *HEAL* DOCUMENTARY

'Dr. David Hamilton is uniquely placed to give compassionate science-backed perspectives on the role that the mind plays in helping to heal the body. In this book, David delves into what we know, whilst making space for what we don't. The world needs more authors – and scientists – like David Hamilton.'
DR. GEMMA NEWMAN, GP AND AUTHOR OF *The Plant Power Doctor*

'As a conscious filmmaker and meditation teacher, I find David's book highly valuable for those scientific nuggets that back up what we know intuitively to be true. He helps us all bridge the gap from woo-woo to, yes, you too!'
ADAM SCHOMER, PRODUCER OF *HEAL* AND *The Road to Dharma*

'Dr. Hamilton has the courage to tackle subjects that are poorly understood and often approached with negative preconceived ideas. He is a true scientist, seeking facts and sharing his understanding with others. I highly recommend this book to anyone interested in improving their own wellness.'
DR. LIZA THOMAS-EMRUS, NHS GP PARTNER AND MEDITATION TEACHER AT REVIVE PRESCRIBED

Why Woo-Woo Works

Also by David R. Hamilton, Ph.D.

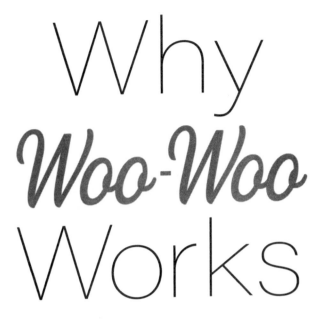

Why Woo-Woo Works

The Surprising Science Behind
Meditation, Reiki, Crystals, and Other
Alternative Practices

David R. Hamilton, Ph.D.

HAY HOUSE

Carlsbad, California • New York City
London • Sydney • New Delhi

Published in the United Kingdom by:
Hay House UK Ltd, The Sixth Floor, Watson House,
54 Baker Street, London W1U 7BU
Tel: +44 (0)20 3927 7290; Fax: +44 (0)20 3927 7291; www.hayhouse.co.uk

Published in the United States of America by:
Hay House Inc., PO Box 5100, Carlsbad, CA 92018-5100
Tel: (1) 760 431 7695 or (800) 654 5126
Fax: (1) 760 431 6948 or (800) 650 5115; www.hayhouse.com

Published in Australia by:
Hay House Australia Pty Ltd, 18/36 Ralph St, Alexandria NSW 2015
Tel: (61) 2 9669 4299; Fax: (61) 2 9669 4144; www.hayhouse.com.au

Published in India by:
Hay House Publishers India, Muskaan Complex,
Plot No.3, B-2, Vasant Kunj, New Delhi 110 070
Tel: (91) 11 4176 1620; Fax: (91) 11 4176 1630; www.hayhouse.co.in

Text © David Hamilton, 2021

The moral rights of the author have been asserted.

The information given in this book should not be treated as a substitute for professional medical advice; always consult a medical practitioner. Any use of information in this book is at the reader's discretion and risk. Neither the author nor the publisher can be held responsible for any loss, claim or damage arising out of the use, or misuse, of the suggestions made, the failure to take medical advice or for any material on third-party websites.

A catalogue record for this book is available from the British Library.

Tradepaper ISBN: 978-1-78817-501-2
E-book ISBN: 978-1-78817-546-3
Audiobook ISBN: 978-1-78817-613-2

Printed and bound by CPI Group (UK) Ltd, Croydon, CR0 4YY

Contents

Introduction

The Oxford University Press's definition of woo-woo is 'Unconventional beliefs regarded as having little or no scientific basis, especially those relating to spirituality, mysticism, or alternative medicine.'[1] The term is believed to have been coined in the 1980s, possibly in imitation of the wailing sound associated with ghosts and the supernatural.

Many complementary therapies, healing modalities, treatments, and other practices, theories, and beliefs are often referred to as woo-woo, but this is because they're not widely understood and most people are unaware that in some instances, they've a sound basis in science.

In the late 1990s, after completing a Ph.D. in organic chemistry, I worked in the pharmaceutical industry, where I helped develop drugs for cardiovascular disease and cancer. Over time, I became fascinated by the fact that in clinical trials, the participants who were given a placebo (a dummy drug) instead of the real drug would very often see an improvement in their condition.

The prevailing belief among scientists was that this phenomenon, which is known as the placebo effect, was some kind of illusion – it wasn't real. My suggestion to colleagues that there might in fact be an effect of the mind on the body – a supposed 'mind–body connection' – was dismissed as quackery.

And yet, even back then, research had shown that expectation (you *will* get better) and belief actually cause biochemical changes in the brain, and this underpins *how* and *why* the placebo effect works. The theory that the mind has an impact on the body wasn't quackery after all. It was supported by scientific evidence. My colleagues and I were just unaware of it at the time.

*****

This is often the case. Science spans a very broad region of knowledge, and it's next to impossible to know everything about every scientific field. Most of us know a lot about one or two things or a small amount about a lot of things. Applying the label woo-woo or pseudoscience to certain beliefs, theories, or practices often betrays our lack of awareness of the available thought or research on them – whether it's from philosophy, psychology, biology, physics, chemistry, geology, cosmology, or other disciplines.

While walking in a park with a friend one day I pointed to a cloud in the sky and told him that it probably weighed around 100 tons (90 tonnes). He laughed – not in an unfriendly way, but just at the preposterous notion that we can establish the weight of a cloud. For him, it conjured up an image of a giant set of kitchen scales. Clearly, it's impossible to know such a thing.

But that's not the case. A cloud is made of water droplets, and to ascertain its weight we can simply fly a drone through it containing a cup of known width and collect water droplets en route. First, the length of the cloud is measured by calculating the time it takes for the drone to fly through it at a given speed, and from there, it's relatively easy to calculate, from the amount of water droplets collected in the cup and the approximate size of the cloud, roughly how much the cloud weighs.

I use this cloud weight example to demonstrate that we often question the veracity of particular theories or ideas simply because we know very little about them, or sometimes even because we've heard other people refer to them as unscientific and it would seem sensible to adopt the same viewpoint. We're social creatures, after all.

In this book I take a number of subjects that are typically denounced as woo-woo and show that there's quite a lot of scientific evidence for them, much of it largely unknown other than to those working in the relevant field.

The first part explores the placebo effect, visualization, meditation, and the link between suppressed emotions and disease. These are at what we might call the 'lower end' of woo-woo in that at least some people are aware of the scientific evidence that exists for them. I share that evidence with you, and also explain exactly *how* these phenomena and practices work.

I then move on to the field of complementary medicine, presenting an overview of the many research studies that show reiki is an effective therapy for managing pain, depression, and anxiety, and sharing the science behind this 'energy healing' technique. In the chapter on crystals, I draw on Buddhist philosophy, the science of color psychology, and even the diamagnetic and paramagnetic properties of these mineral stones to explain precisely *how* they work for us.

In the latter part of the book I delve into telepathy, distant healing, and prayer. Although these phenomena are often dismissed as pseudoscience, there is in fact a large amount of statistical evidence to support them, although it's not widely known to the general public. As we'll discuss, one of the key factors in the way they work is emotional connection: EEG and MRI studies show that the more emotionally connected two people are, the stronger any effects tend to be.

*****

My interest in esoteric topics began when I was a child. My mum developed postpartum (postnatal) depression in 1976, following the birth of the youngest of my three sisters. The condition wasn't well understood at that time – 'Give yourself a shake,' was one doctor's recommendation.

She was prescribed antidepressants and antianxiety medication, but the thing that worked best for her was meditation. It didn't cure her, but it helped her get to sleep, enabled her to better manage her state, and supported her mind and emotions through difficult times.

My mum's practice was listening to a guided meditation tape every night before bed, and she continued with it for years because it worked so well. The tape featured relaxing music and the sounds of nature, which, as we'll explore in the book, are now known to have a direct impact on the human autonomic nervous system.

Meditation has long been practiced in cultures around the world and yet it was considered pseudoscience in the West until fairly recently; in some places, that's still the case. However, today we know with scientific certainty that meditation causes beneficial structural changes in the brain that help us with our mental health as well as with concentration, memory, and self-esteem – it's even been shown to slow the rate of biological aging.

While I was growing up, my mum and I talked often about the power of the mind, and this shared interest, and my observation that it had helped her condition, led to my fascination with the placebo effect when I worked in the pharmaceutical industry.

In the years since, and even today, mum and I have had many more conversations about these and other 'woo-woo' subjects – many of which are covered in this book – and eventually these catalyzed a career change for me. I left the pharmaceutical industry and went on to write several books exploring the mind–body connection, self-esteem, and even the impact of kindness on mental and physical health.

In this book, I present the science behind woo-woo and reveal how and why it really works. I hope you enjoy it.

Dr. David R. Hamilton
March, 2021

CHAPTER 1

Mind Over Matter

'They're *not* getting better. They just *think* they're getting better.' This was a typical sentiment expressed by my pharmaceutical company colleagues when I asked for their opinion of the placebo effect, a phenomenon that was particularly relevant to our work given that the drugs we were developing would be tested in clinical trials.

This view was always offered amicably, but it underlined the assumption, held for decades, that the placebo effect was 'all in the mind.' If a patient who had been given a placebo in a drugs trial got better, it was written off as part of the natural course of their illness – it would have happened anyway.

A placebo is an inactive (or dummy) treatment, in the form of a pill, injection, or device, that's administered in clinical trials to test the real drug or treatment against a control (comparison). As such, a placebo isn't designed to have any therapeutic effects on the patients who take it. However, in reality, it often does – and when this happens it's because the patients believe the placebo is the real drug or treatment: it's their *belief* that does the work.

Belief Alters Biology

The placebo effect might appear to be an illusion, but science has shown that belief itself has real biological effects. Admittedly, this does sound a bit woo-woo; however, woo-woo is only woo-woo in our mind until we know the science, and then it's 'true woo.'

> *In fact, there's no question that belief causes chemical changes in the brain, and these changes are dependent on what a person believes.*

For example, patients can believe opposite things about the same placebo and get opposite effects from it. If a patient believes that a pill (if it's a placebo) will *reduce* pain, it *will* usually reduce pain. Yet if they had believed it would *cause* pain it would have done that instead. In the former case, the belief causes the production of the brain's natural versions of morphine.

In the USA, scientists at the University of California at San Francisco showed that endogenous opioids, the brain's own morphine, were responsible for the painkilling effects of placebos used during dental surgery.[1] But crucially, the endogenous opioids are produced in response to a person's belief or expectation that the pain will go away. If a patient believes that a pill (if it's a placebo) will cause pain, the belief *blocks* these natural opioids in the brain, essentially elevating pain.[2]

A belief that a pill (if it's a placebo) will help us relax will bring about a calming effect, yet if we believe that it's a stimulant, we'll feel agitated and our heart rate and blood pressure will rise – even though, in both cases, the pill is a dummy.

When a group of athletes were given substances that they believed would increase their strength and endurance, they did indeed gain strength and endurance. But the substances were placebos. Luckily, these 'performance-enhancing placebos' (PEPs) couldn't get them banned from competition because they were, well, dummies. Perhaps many athletes just need a PEP talk.[3]

And in research conducted by scientists in the departments of psychiatry and medicine at the State University of New York, 40 patients with either asthma, emphysema, or restrictive lung disease were given an inhaler containing a nebulized saline placebo but were told that it contained allergens that would restrict their airways.[4] Before long, 19 of the patients reacted with considerable constriction of their airways. Twelve, in fact, had a full asthma attack. When they were given a different inhaler and told it would relieve their symptoms, even though it was also a saline placebo, it did relieve their symptoms.

Therefore, that one placebo inhaler either reduced or created bronchospasm in asthma sufferers, depending on what the patients *believed* it would do. One person even developed symptoms of hay fever when they were told that the inhaler also contained pollen, and those symptoms were again relieved when they were given another saline inhaler that they believed would do that.

Studying the Placebo Effect

It's also possible to use color as a placebo because of what it represents to us. In the USA, in a unique way of teaching medical students about the placebo effect, University of Cincinnati medical professors gave a class of students pink and blue placebo pills and told them that they were stimulants and sedatives.[5] It was found that the blue pills were 66 percent effective as sedatives, compared with 26 percent for the pink pills.

In other words, blue placebos were around two and a half times better than pink ones for helping people to relax. This is because for most people, blue is a calming color, and this informs some of what we believe it will do. The researchers also found that giving the students two placebos rather than one was more effective.

And as strange as it sounds, although perhaps not to parents, for children, a plaster illustrated with a colorful cartoon or a magical character reduces pain and heals a cut faster than a plain plaster.[6]

Where we live also affects the power of a placebo. In a US study of migraine treatments, placebo injections were found to be 1.5 times more powerful than placebo pills, while a European trial found that placebo pills were about 10 percent more effective than placebo injections.[7]

The reason for the difference lies in our cultural language. Americans tend to speak of 'getting a shot,' so they're more likely to believe in injections, whereas Europeans talk of 'popping pills' (or at least they do in the UK), so they place their faith in pills.

In a similar way, in trials of Tagamet, an anti-ulcer drug popular in the 1970s and 80s, the placebo was 59 percent effective in France but the drug itself was 60 percent effective in Brazil.[8] Advertising budgets for drugs are higher in Western Europe than in South America, and more advertising spending creates a stronger perception of the power of a drug, but it has the same effect on the placebo.

Perception Matters

The way a placebo is packaged also makes a difference to its power. In a study at Keele University in the UK, 835 women were given one of four different pills for headache.[9] One group received a well-known branded aspirin tablet, while a second group received an aspirin tablet simply labeled 'analgesic,' which was typical of a cheaper mass-market brand. A third group received a branded placebo labeled 'aspirin,' while a fourth group took a basic unbranded placebo that was labeled 'analgesic.'

It transpired that the branded aspirin worked better than the unbranded one, and the main difference was in the appearance of the packaging; however, amazingly, the branded placebo worked better than the unbranded placebo – even though they were both made of sugar.

This explains why so many people swear that branded painkillers such as Nurofen (Advil) work better for them than generic packs of ibuprofen, even though they contain the same drug. There's a significant price difference and Nurofen has more expensive-looking packaging, so people expect more from it. Drugs are designed to carry out a biological function, but as well as the impact of a drug on the body, the *mind* also has an impact.

You might now see why for most people, an expensive drug works better than a cheaper one. The same might also be true of a more expensive therapist. But what really makes both better – the drug and the therapist – is the person's mind.

Perception is important, even when we're not consciously aware of the contents of our mind.

According to a paper published in *Advances in Psychiatric Treatment*, this might even enhance the power of the drug Viagra, which is used to treat erectile dysfunction, beyond its basic pharmacological effect.[10] The name 'Viagra' sounds similar to the words 'vigor' and 'Niagara,' and given that Niagara Falls is a *force of nature*, this might create a perception of vigorousness and natural power. I wonder if the drug would work so well if it was called 'Softy'!

The Power of Positive Consultation

In some cases, the mind can *enhance* the effects of a drug – depending on what the patient believes it's supposed to do, or on their perception of the doctor who prescribed it – and in other cases it can *suppress* the effects, in accordance with what they believe.

We know this because some of the variation in the placebo effect simply comes down to communication between medical staff and patients. For relatively common ailments, a doctor who shows confidence or optimism about the patient's recovery is much more likely to see them get better than one who is unsure or pessimistic.

For example, based on studies that show that no firm diagnosis is made for about 40–60 percent of patients visiting general practice surgeries (offices), a University of Southampton study in the UK investigated the consequences of different styles of consultation in patients in this category.

Publishing in the *British Medical Journal*, they compared the outcomes of 200 patients, half of whom received a consultation that was conducted in a 'positive' manner while the other half received a consultation that was conducted in a 'non-positive' manner.[11]

In the 'positive' consultations, the patients were given a firm diagnosis and confidently told that they would recover in a few days' time. Sometimes a prescription was given and the doctor assured the patient that it would make them better; at other times, no prescription was given and the doctor assured the patient that none was needed.

In the 'non-positive' consultations, the doctor displayed uncertainty, saying, 'I cannot be certain what is the matter with you.' If the doctor was offering a treatment, they would add, 'I'm not sure that the treatment I'm going to give you will have an effect.' If no treatment was to be given, the doctor would instead add, 'and therefore I will give you no treatment.'

The prescription given for those patients being treated was 3 mg of vitamin B1, marked 'thiamine hydrochloride,' a very low dose that was essentially a placebo. After two weeks, 64 percent of the patients who had received the positive consultation were better, compared with only 39 percent of the patients who had recovered after receiving a non-positive consultation. And it didn't matter whether they were treated or not. The difference in how many patients recovered, almost double, was down to the way the doctor communicated with the patient.

Why does belief cause these effects? Painkilling placebos work because the person *expects* to feel a reduction in pain. This expectation causes their brain to produce its own natural painkillers, which then reduce the pain.

Studies at the Neurodegenerative Disorders Center at the University of British Columbia in Canada have shown that believing a placebo is an anti-Parkinson's drug causes the brain to produce the neurotransmitter dopamine.[12] Here, and in the case of painkilling effects, belief mobilizes the brain's natural resources to meet the person's expectations. That is, a belief about what's supposed to happen instructs the brain to produce what it needs to produce to deliver that result.

Of course, this applies only within reason. Belief that a placebo is a chemotherapy drug doesn't make the brain produce its own chemotherapy drug, and there could never be an ethical case to experiment with this. However, some documented spontaneous remissions in patients may have occurred because belief, or faith, mobilized the immune system.

Can We Harness the Placebo Effect?

In the department of cardiovascular surgery at the Heart Center of the University of Marburg in Germany, 124 patients scheduled for coronary artery bypass graft surgery were randomly distributed into three groups.

The first was the 'Expect' group, where the focus was on optimizing patients' positive expectations of life after surgery, such as engaging in activities; the second was the 'Support' group, where patients received emotional support; and the third was the 'Standard medical care' group, where patients received the usual treatment.[13]

Patients were followed for six months after their surgery. Those in the 'Expect' group had much greater quality of life and subjective working ability than those in the other two groups. Support was helpful too, but expecting that things would go well had by far the greatest effect. When doctors give hope to patients, helping them to *expect* to get better, they *do* get better faster.

Placebo-Controlled Dose Reduction

An exciting line of research into harnessing the placebo effect is placebo-controlled dose reduction (PCDR), where scientists give a drug for a few days and then, without the patients' knowledge, swap it for a placebo. The more times the patients receive the drug, the more strongly they associate relief of symptoms with receiving the drug, and so the stronger is the effect of the placebo when the swap is made. In this way, the dose of a drug can be reduced and replaced by a placebo.

Fabrizio Benedetti, Professor of Physiology and Neuroscience at the University of Turin Medical School in Italy, powerfully demonstrated this effect with a study involving Parkinson's disease patients.[14]

The patients were split into several groups. All but one group received a full dose of the anti-Parkinson's drug apomorphine on day 1 of the study, and Benedetti measured their clinical response as a reduction in tremors and muscle stiffness and also in the degree of activation of individual neurons in the brain region known to be affected by the condition. He gave the other group a placebo injection (saline) instead, and there was no clinical effect whatsoever.

Over the next few days, Benedetti swapped the drug for the placebo in different groups. One group who got the drug on day 1 received the placebo on day 2. Another group received the drug for two days and it was swapped for the placebo on the third day, and yet another group received the drug for three days before it was swapped for the placebo on day 4.

Each time a patient received a dose of apomorphine, they had the experience of 'when I receive this injection, my tremors reduce and my muscle stiffness lessens,' and each day, the effect of the placebo became stronger.

On day 5, Benedetti did the drug-placebo swap for the final group, who had received apomorphine on the previous four days. They had built up even more of the experience of 'when I receive this injection, my tremors reduce and my muscle stiffness lessens.'

Amazingly, the strength of the saline placebo matched that of the drug, reducing tremors and muscle stiffness and activating neurons to the same degree. Benedetti reported, 'It should be noted that placebo administration following four apomorphine preconditioning trials induced clinical responses that were as large as those to apomorphine.'

Some patients were initially given a placebo to see if it had any effects, and there were none. Yet, after four days of experience of associating the drug with a change in symptoms, the drug could be phased out and replaced with a placebo. These results weren't just 'all in the mind' because there were measurable changes in the brain in the striatum – the region that's usually deficient in dopamine in Parkinson's patients.

The same kind of effect seen with placebo-controlled dose reduction has also been demonstrated with the immune system, where a phased swapping of an immunosuppressant drug (cyclosporin A) for a placebo suppressed the immune system.[15] PCDR works because expectation and belief cause physical changes in biochemistry.

The aim of this line of research on the immune system is to help patients receiving organ transplants, or even those with autoimmune conditions such as multiple sclerosis (MS), rheumatoid arthritis, and lupus. Ultimately, if PCDR could be applied to a larger range of medical conditions, it could result in a huge cost saving, allowing funds to be funneled into other areas of healthcare.

PCDR may also reduce the side effects of medication. In one PCDR study, children with ADHD had 50 percent of their drug dose swapped with placebo and there was evidence that they experienced fewer stimulant-related side effects.[16]

The Nocebo Effect

It's sometimes the case that people experience side effects with placebos, when they know what the side effects are. This is known as the nocebo effect. While the word placebo is derived from the Latin for 'I shall please,' the word nocebo comes from 'I shall harm.' It's where the *expectation* of a negative effect produces one.

A randomized controlled trial (RCT) is a clinical trial in which patients are randomly assigned – selected by chance – to receive a drug or placebo, and neither the patient nor the research team knows who receives what. In Greece, a statistical analysis of 21 randomized controlled trials of antidepressants conducted at the neurology department of Athens Naval Hospital and the First Psychiatric Department of Eginition University Hospital found that about 45 percent of patients who received placebos reported the side effects of nausea, headache, and dizziness, which were the expected side effects of the drug itself.[17]

In another statistical study of 56 studies, 74 percent of MS patients experienced side effects after receiving placebos.[18] And in a study conducted by Bayer Pharmaceuticals that examined drug and placebo treatments for patients with angina or diabetes, researchers found that the side effect profile for the placebo was largely the same as that for the drug.[19]

Typically, if a person knows what the side effects of a drug are, they get those side effects when they receive a placebo – *provided* they're unaware that they're taking a placebo. However, if they don't know what the side effects of a drug are, they don't typically get them.

The Expectation of Better

I sometimes refer to the placebo effect as the perception effect. One reason for this is that many people still consider a placebo to be empty – any seeming improvement in the patient who receives one must be a figment of their imagination. As we've discussed, for years, the idea that belief could impact biology was considered woo-woo.

However, we now know with factual certainty that chemical changes occur in the body when a person believes that a placebo is a real drug. With placebo painkillers, people experience less pain. They aren't imagining it – their pain *really is* less, and that's down to the natural painkillers that are produced in their brain because they believe the placebo is a painkiller.

As I mentioned earlier, more expensive-looking placebos are more effective at reducing pain than cheaper-looking ones; the fancier packaging creates the *perception* that the placebo is better, so patients expect more from it.

As a culture, we've agreed on the story that if one thing is more expensive than another, then it must also be *better*. We've heard it many times in our lives and we've also had direct experience of it – most of us tend to get more wear out of a more expensive jacket or pair of shoes, say, than our everyday inexpensive clothing.

So when we pay more for the same medicine or treatment, our expectation of *better* generally makes it so for us. Of course, this applies within reason, and I'm not condoning the use of highly expensive unproven treatments that sometimes cost people their life savings. I'm referring in general to the fact that our beliefs and perception alter our brain and body biochemistry in a direction that confirms what we believe is supposed to happen.

Biology will always follow perception. When perception shifts, so does biology. In one study, for example, volunteers were shown an image of a horrific car accident in which people had sustained serious injuries. There was a massive spike in the volunteers' nervous systems as their bodies reacted with stress to the image.

However, they were then reassured that the image wasn't of a real accident: it was a still from a movie set, and the apparently injured people were actors wearing makeup for the scene. Almost instantaneously, the volunteers' nervous systems calmed. They didn't just feel calmer in their mind – there was a significant physiological effect that followed from their perceptions.

The Power of Our Imagination

To a large extent, the brain doesn't distinguish real from imaginary, and this underpins some aspects of the placebo effect. When you imagine that something is happening, it really is happening as far as your brain in concerned, and it releases the chemical substances necessary to confirm that what you're imagining is indeed real.

One of my favorite scientific studies is affectionately known as the piano study.[20] In 1995, Alvaro Pascual-Leone, a professor of neurology at Harvard Medical School in the USA, asked a group of volunteers to play a sequence of five notes on a piano every day for five days. Each session involved playing notes for two hours, one note with each finger of the hand, moving up and down a scale of five notes.

While the volunteers did this, a separate group did the same thing, only without a piano. They closed their eyes and *imagined* that they were playing the five notes in this way. This is called kinesthetic imagery, and it's where we re-create movement by vividly imagining how it feels to move.

Each volunteer had a daily brain scan, and at the end of the five days, those who had played the notes on the piano had considerable changes in the brain region connected to their finger muscles; however, the same was true of the volunteers who had imagined playing the notes. In fact, on comparing the scans, it wasn't possible to tell whether a scan came from a person who had played the notes with their fingers or with their mind.

Visualization to Enhance Performance

It was already known at the time of the piano study that athletes could enhance their performance by practicing visualization, but this was the first brain-imaging confirmation of what's actually happening when a person visualizes something. The prevailing belief among sports coaches was that visualization worked by enhancing an athlete's focus and their motivation to train and practice. Any notion that the brain was actually changing was swiftly dismissed as pseudoscience.

In the mid to late 1990s, I served as a part-time athletics coach and manager of the junior (under 20s) men's team of a large and very successful athletics club in Manchester in the UK. I also competed myself as a long jumper.

One day at a junior athletics event, a PE teacher told me about the time she met Ed Moses, the former 400 meters hurdles men's world record holder and multiple world and Olympic gold medalist. The great American athlete had been in the UK for an international competition and he'd visited her school to speak to the children about sports.

The following day at the meeting, the teacher watched as Moses' fellow athletes warmed up before the race, stretching and striding up and down the track, but she couldn't see him anywhere. She eventually spotted him lying down beside a hurdle, with his eyes closed. She wondered what on earth he was doing, seemingly losing valuable warm-up time.

Shortly before the race, Moses got up, did some stretches and a few sprints, and then went out and won, a good 30 feet (10 meters) clear of the other runners. The teacher had a chance to chat with him afterward and asked him if he'd been doing some kind of relaxation exercise beforehand, or if he'd even been asleep.

Moses explained that he'd been visualizing. He'd imagined the whole race in his mind – from the moment the starting pistol fired to reaching the first hurdle, and the feelings and sensations in his body as he cleared it; then taking exactly 13 strides to the next hurdle before clearing that too, and so on. He'd pictured himself running the race in the way he wanted to run it.

A few years later, I met the British athlete Sally Gunnell, also a former world and Olympic gold medalist and 400 meters hurdles women's world record holder, at a corporate event at which we were both speaking. Afterward, we chatted about visualization, because Sally had explained to the audience that 70 percent of winning an Olympic gold medal is mental, and that a large amount of her personal practice was visualization.

Like Moses, Gunnell visualized running the whole race, stride for stride, hurdle for hurdle, but with particular focus on the last portion; in a 400 meters hurdles race, this is the stage at which athletes often feel that their legs are as heavy as lead. When she visualized this part of the race, Gunnell would imagine her legs feeling light and moving with ease; she would repetitively visualize running in a relaxed way, even if another athlete appeared to be catching up with her, something that typically causes athletes to tense up.

Gunnell explained that she'd started doing visualization work after finishing a disappointing sixth at the 1990 European Championships. When she won the Olympic 400 meters hurdles title in 1992, and broke the world record at the World Championships the following year, she was reaping great rewards from her mental practice.

Practice Plus Visualization

While I worked in the pharmaceutical industry and coached and competed in athletics on the side, I shared with a few colleagues that I was experimenting with visualization practice. Most were supportive, but some found it amusing that, as a scientist, I was working with techniques widely regarded as pseudoscience. It was friendly banter, but typical of the assumption at the time.

I continued to practice all the same, but kept it to myself. In a three-month experiment, I practiced visualization almost daily, and I also listened to a Paul McKenna 'Ultimate Athlete' self-hypnosis tape, which helped me to believe in myself. And in an outcome that I found astonishing myself, my long jump personal best improved by almost 3 feet (1 meter). The improvement was significant enough for me to recognize just how effective visualization could be, even in a short time, long before I became aware of the neuroscience research.

> **Visualization does more than improve an athlete's focus and motivation – it also affects their brain networks and significantly alters the strength and movement range of their muscles.**

In multiple studies, scientists have compared the strength of people lifting weights with people *imagining* lifting weights and have found relatively small differences in strength between the 'real' and 'imaginary' groups.

One study by researchers in the department of biomedical engineering at the Lerner Research Institute in Cleveland, USA, for example, compared volunteers flexing a finger several times a day with volunteers imagining flexing the finger, and found that while those who did the real movement increased their finger strength by 53 percent, those who did no movement but just imagined it increased their strength by 35 percent.[21]

Following copious amounts of modern research, it's now well understood that the optimum way to enhance performance in any sport or movement is to combine physical practice with visualization. In order of best first, research shows that physical practice plus visualization is more effective than physical practice alone, which is better than visualization practice alone.

Visualization to Assist Recovery

The aforementioned kind of practice has also helped hundreds of people to recover faster after suffering a stroke. In multiple research studies, stroke patients received either standard physiotherapy or physiotherapy plus visualization, and those who did visualization in addition to their physiotherapy improved to a greater degree and much faster than those who did physiotherapy alone.

For example, in a University of Cincinnati study in the department of physical medicine and rehabilitation, after each physiotherapy session, chronic stroke patients listened to a tape that guided them through visualizations of moving the hand, arm, and shoulder of their impaired side.[22] When tested after six weeks, the patients' arm function was significantly better than that of patients in a control group who did relaxation after physiotherapy.

A large meta-analysis has since referred to visualization as a 'viable intervention' for people recovering from a stroke.[23] And yet 20 years ago, visualization was still considered pseudoscience.

Further analyses suggest that in some stroke patients, visualization even helps repair some damaged brain regions, and in some others the area responsible for movement switches to a new brain location that isn't damaged, permitting neuroplasticity there and a return to more able movements. In one neurological study, for example, researchers reported that the brains of stroke patients who used visualization had undergone some degree of cortical reorganization as a consequence of their mental practice.[24]

Thinking Kindness

The real versus imaginary phenomenon is much more widespread than in the areas we've discussed so far, though. The brain produces stress hormones regardless of whether we're in a stressful situation or *imagining* a stressful situation. It's the feelings of stress that trigger the release of stress hormones such as adrenaline and cortisol, independently of the situation itself.

For example, two friends are sitting in a car that's stuck in traffic. One feels stressed at the thought of being late for her appointment, while the other accepts the situation: she knows that she can't do much about it, so she relaxes. The first woman will have elevated levels of the stress hormones cortisol and adrenaline. The second won't. Do these levels have anything to do with the situation itself? Not so much. They've more to do with how each individual *feels* about the situation.

The same kind of thing happens with kindness. As I explored in my books *The Five Side Effects of Kindness* and *The Little Book of Kindness*, the opposite of the feeling of stress is the feeling induced by kindness.[25] Most of us assume that the opposite of stress is peace, calm, or a feeling of relaxation, but these states represent the absence of stress, not its opposite.

In research that recorded people's daily stress score and the approximate number of kind things said or done, stress and kindness sat opposite each other: as if on a see-saw, as kindness went up, stress came down, and vice versa. It didn't mean that kindness causes an absence of stressful events, only that both feelings can't coexist and so as we increase feelings induced by kindness, these take some of the sting out of normally stressful events. Therefore, if you want to reduce stress, try kindness.

Kindness Hormones

Just as feelings of stress produce stress hormones, kindness has its own biological products. I call these kindness hormones in my books and blogs, to point out that they're produced by *feelings*, just as stress hormones are.

The main kindness hormone is oxytocin. Well known for its importance in reproduction, breast feeding, and even social bonding, and occasionally going by such affectionate names as the love drug, the hugging hormone, and even the cuddle chemical, oxytocin also plays a considerable number of other key roles in the body.

Oxytocin protects the cardiovascular system, and just as stress hormones increase blood pressure, this kindness hormone lowers it. It also has antioxidant and anti-inflammatory properties, helps with digestion and wound healing, and is even involved in the construction of heart muscle and many other cell types from stem cells.

At around 500 million years old, the oxytocin gene is one of the oldest in the human genome, and during that time, it has integrated into many important functions in the human body. What this means is that all of these functions are impacted by how kindness *feels*, just as many functions in the brain and body are impacted by how stress feels.

Most prior work in this area of research has charted the course of stress through the brain and body. We're only now beginning to examine the side effects of positive feelings, and they're plentiful. Psychologically, positive feelings increase happiness, build resilience, and protect against depression. They impact brain function and even cause neurological changes if they're experienced over a period of time; they also reduce inflammation and even help us to live longer.

Both positive and negative feelings can be induced in a real situation or an imagined one. Just as your brain doesn't distinguish between a real stressful event and an imagined one, it's the same with kindness.

> *Your brain will produce kindness hormones when you're being kind, witnessing an act of kindness, imagining one, or even recalling one.*

In each case, you feel how kindness feels and your feelings trigger the physiological effects as a consequence. Thinking of things that annoy us fuels feelings of stress, and subsequently the physiology of stress. Thinking kindness does the opposite – thinking kind things about people, which *generates* kind feelings, can be a simple way to reduce stress.

More Visualization Studies

Carey Morewedge, then at Carnegie Mellon University in the USA, invited volunteers to eat sweets or cubes of cheese and others to imagine eating the sweets or cheese.[26] He found that real and imagined eating impacted appetite in more or less the same way.

Just as eating food gradually reduces appetite by activating specific brain regions – otherwise we'd never stop – imagining eating seemed to have the same effect. Morewedge reported that research is revealing that the division between real and imaginary, as far as the brain is concerned, is becoming increasingly blurred.

It's important to be aware that the volunteers in this study had to imagine the *entire* process of eating. Making a quick mental picture of the sweet or cheese wouldn't work: they had to imagine picking up the food and chewing it in the same way they would if they really were eating it – bite for bite, chew for chew. If they'd usually chew 10 times before swallowing, they had to imagine chewing 10 times before imagining swallowing.

Even the immune system responds to the imagination. Following research in which volunteers were able to increase immune system antibodies by visualizing their increase, researchers at the United Lincolnshire Hospitals NHS Trust in the UK conducted a randomized controlled trial of women receiving treatment for breast cancer.[27]

All of the women received their normal scheduled treatment (chemotherapy, surgery, radiotherapy, and hormone therapy), but half also did daily visualization sessions. Each woman randomized to the visualization group visualized her immune system destroying cancer cells. Many imagined their immune cells as piranha fish or even as a Pac-Man character. Some visualized macrophages gobbling cancer cells.

The women who visualized were found to have much higher levels of key immune cells, such as natural killer (NK) cells, T cells, and T helper cells, than those who didn't visualize, and this was even after four cycles of chemotherapy. Publishing in the respected journal *The Breast*, researchers reported that the immune system was still showing high cytotoxicity against cancer cells after the four cycles, but only in the women who were visualizing their immune cells destroying cancer cells.

Positive Affirmations

The key to making visualization work is repetition, which has been shown to impact brain networks, shaping them in the direction of producing what it is we're imagining. My first experience of this kind of repetition was positive affirmations, which do something similar. The *Psychology Dictionary* defines an affirmation as 'a brief phase which is spoken again and again in an effort to plant seeds of happy and positive notions, conceptions, and attitudes into one's psyche.'[28]

In the late 19th century, the French psychologist Émile Coué noted that his patients often recovered faster if he helped them to expect to get better. So he developed what he called autosuggestions, the best known of which is 'Every day, in every way, I'm getting better and better.'

Nowadays we refer to autosuggestions as positive affirmations, or as positive self-affirmations when they affirm our core values. They help us to think and feel more positive and, as a consequence, take positive affirmative action.

Serious research into affirmations began in the 1980s, when the American social psychologist Claude Steele published a paper on his self-affirmation theory.[29] This posits that humans are fundamentally motivated to maintain a positive self-view – that is, a general perception of ourselves as good, virtuous, competent, stable, capable of free choice, and as having a sense of control over important outcomes in our lives.

Self-affirmations, then, are statements that affirm our core values; for example, if one has a core value of kindness, the affirmation would be something like: 'I am a good person.' Research has shown that when we state something that affirms our values in this way, it makes us think and feel more positive; we're also much more likely to indulge in healthy behaviors and are more likely to take positive steps to improve our lives. This is especially the case when affirmations are repeated.

Changing Our Behavior for the Better

A study by scientists at the University of Pennsylvania in the USA showed that this may be because repeating affirmations produces physical changes in specific brain regions associated with self-processing.[30] Repeating affirmations didn't just make the volunteers feel a little better or more positive in the moment, it actually altered brain networks that essentially wired in the feeling. And those brain changes were found to account for a subsequent change in the volunteers' behavior.

A collaboration between scientists at the universities of Aston, Sussex, and King's College London, published in the *Journal of Sport and Exercise Psychology*, examined the effect of self-affirmations on healthy behavior.[31] They enlisted 80 volunteers, half of whom were randomized to work on self-affirmations, while the other half were in a control group.

The volunteers wrote self-affirmations based on their most important personal values. They were then shown a fact sheet that outlined the benefits of exercise, such as improved mood and better health, as well as the risks of a sedentary lifestyle, such as an increased risk of heart disease.

When followed up just one week later, the volunteers who did the self-affirmations were undertaking significantly more physical activity, had more positive attitudes toward exercise, and had higher intentions to exercise than those in the control group, who hadn't done any affirmations.

A study at the University of Sheffield in the UK found that changes in healthy behavior applied to diet too.[32] Ninety-three women were randomized either to write self-affirmations or be in a control group. They were then shown information about the health benefits of eating fruits and vegetables. Over a week, those women who did the self-affirmations ate, on average, 5.5 more portions of fruits and vegetables than those who didn't do the affirmations.

Research has also shown that self-affirmations can be very helpful for those times in our lives when challenges and threats can seem like mountains to climb – which is essentially what Émile Coué's affirmation was designed to do.

Self-affirmations can help us to overcome stress and make gradual improvements in our lives and in our health.

According to psychologists at UC Santa Barbara and Cornell University, this is because self-affirmations help us to expand and broaden our sense of self, while at the same time making a challenge or threat seem smaller.[33] It's a relative shift: affirmations make us feel bigger and the threat or challenge seems smaller as a consequence.

Affirmations were greatly popularized from the 1980s onward by Louise Hay, one of the founders of the self-help movement, who had noted that many of her therapy clients who presented with the same symptoms or conditions had a similar attitude or way of thinking about themselves. She often gave them positive affirmations, as Coué did, which helped steer their thinking in a healthier direction. Many of these affirmations can be found in Hay's book *You Can Heal Your Life*.

CHAPTER 2

Meditation

My initial perception of meditation, before it became a key part of my personal practice, was of bare-chested Indian gurus repeatedly chanting the syllable *om*. *Om* is the best-known example of a mantra, which is similar to an affirmation.

The word mantra is derived from two Sanskrit words: *manas* (mind) and *tra* (tools or instruments) – literally a mind tool. In the Hindu and Buddhist traditions, a mantra is a sound, a word, or a short phase that's intoned repeatedly during meditation, contemplation, or prayer – a technique that's been practiced for thousands of years.

Mantra-Based Meditation

A key difference between an affirmation and a mantra is that while the former tends to be a positive statement, the latter is a mystical utterance that's considered sacred and to have deep spiritual significance. In Hinduism and Buddhism, *om* is the most sacred of all the mantras; it refers to Atman (which is soul or the self within) and Brahman (ultimate reality, truth, universe, divine, supreme being). Mystics say that the sound produces vibrations in our consciousness that align us with universal consciousness.

Many mantras are words or phrases associated with love or compassion, or are statements of spiritual insight. For example, the most widely used mantra in Buddhism, *Om mani padme hum*, translates to 'the jewel is in the lotus' and implies that if we follow and practice a good path, we can transform our impure mind into the pure mind of a Buddha.

Another key difference between an affirmation and a mantra is that an affirmation tends to require a determined mental effort to make a focused statement, while a mantra requires much less effort – it's more passive and has a calming effect. This is evidenced by brain-imaging studies; while affirmations tend to activate brain regions associated with concentration, mantras tend to deactivate and calm these regions.

> *Mantra-based meditation can be*
> *extremely relaxing and is effective for*
> *counteracting worry and stress.*

For example, in 2015, scientists at the Weizmann Institute of Science in Rehovot, Israel, examined the brain activity of non-meditators who were invited to repeat the simple mantra 'One' (*echad* in Hebrew). They found that repeating the mantra quieted brain activity in regions of the brain involved in mental chatter and self-judgment.[1]

Transcendental Meditation (TM), which was introduced to the West in the mid-1950s by Maharishi Mahesh Yogi, is a popular mantra-based meditation technique that's typically practiced twice daily for 15–20 minutes. Numerous studies attest to TM's ability to produce relaxing states, and effects that follow from those states.

For example, a 2019 randomized controlled study of 40 teaching and support staff at a US school for students with severe behavioral problems – who had reported various degrees of workplace stress and burnout – showed that a twice-daily practice of TM significantly reduced their stress levels over a four-month period of practice.[2]

In 2013, the American Heart Association stated that TM is a beneficial treatment for hypertension, while a 2015 review and meta-analysis conducted by researchers at Lanzhou University's Evidence-Based Medicine Center in China concluded that a practice of TM could reduce blood pressure.[3]

As well as reducing negative mental chatter, calming the mind, and promoting better mental and physical health, the use of mantra-based meditation has even helped some people to attain mystical states of consciousness.

Mindfulness Meditation

Many popular meditation techniques don't use mantras; instead, like the widely practiced mindfulness, they simply invite us to bring our attention to our breath. We all breathe, but if we do so while *noticing* that we're breathing – giving our attention for a moment or two to what it sounds like to breathe, what it feels like to breathe – we're meditating. We're being *mindful* of the fact that we're breathing; this practice is often called mindfulness.

When I first tried mindfulness meditation in the late 1990s, while working as a scientist in the pharmaceutical industry, I kept it from my friends and colleagues in order to protect my professional reputation. Back then, the practice was considered spiritual mumbo jumbo, and papers had been published warning doctors not to recommend it to patients, lest they be considered quacks.

Today, meditation, including mindfulness, is widely accepted in the scientific and corporate worlds, and with the general public. Many CEOs practice it and some have even created dedicated meditation rooms in their businesses. I've personally taught meditation to sales and customer service staff and even to senior police officers.

> *Meditation is an example of how a mystical practice becomes mainstream once the science is known and enough people are doing it.*

Over and above the reported effects of mantra-based practices, meditation has more far-reaching benefits. It's been shown to help people deal with anxiety and stress, and the reason for this is that meditating changes the physical structure of the brain. When we repeatedly practice mindfulness and notice our breath, we 'exercise' the dorsolateral prefrontal cortex – which is the 'noticing' part of the brain – as well as a few other brain regions. It's almost as if we're taking it to the gym.

Working Out the Brain

When we work on a muscle in the gym, it becomes both firmer and larger. And as a result of neuroplasticity – the ability of the brain to adapt to its environment and change with experience – something similar occurs when we 'work out' a brain region. It becomes firmer – denser in neural connections, akin to muscle fibers – and larger, in that it occupies a greater volume.

And, just as repeatedly exercising a muscle makes it more powerful, and everything for which we use it becomes easier, so working out a region of the brain makes it more powerful, and everything for which it's used becomes easier.

The dorsolateral prefrontal cortex is the area of the brain involved in self-control, our ability to manage our state, and concentration, and it also plays a role in the experience of positive emotional states like happiness and joy. So, when we work out the dorsolateral prefrontal cortex through mindfulness practice, we become more in control of ourselves, better able to manage our mental and emotional state, and find it easier to access happiness. Numerous scientific studies have confirmed this.

However, there comes a point when, through sustained meditation practice over several years, that activation in the brain's attention areas begins to decrease; this occurs to such a degree that advanced practitioners show less activation there than do novice practitioners. While studying the brains of advanced meditation practitioners, researchers at the University of Wisconsin in the USA showed that they had developed the ability to be acutely focused with hardly any effort, just as an advanced tennis player or golfer develops the ability to play at the highest level with seemingly minimal effort.[4]

Loving-Kindness Meditation

Different types of meditation work out different regions of the brain. Instead of mindfulness, we can try a practice I refer to as *kindfulness* – which is similar to mindfulness, but with thoughts and sentiments of kindness and compassion added to the mix.

An example of kindfulness practice is the Buddhist style known as loving-kindness meditation (also referred to as *metta*), which is thought of as an unselfish desire to help someone who is suffering. As well as an awareness of the breath, loving-kindness meditation builds a sentiment of love, compassion, and kindness. A typical loving-kindness practice is: 'May you be happy. May you be well. May you be safe. May you be at ease.'

The subject of a loving-kindness meditation changes – focusing at times on ourselves, on our loved ones, on friends, neighbors, work colleagues, even difficult people, and all sentient beings – but the sentiment of love, kindness, and compassion is present throughout.

Scientific studies have shown that this type of practice works out the regions of the brain associated with empathy, compassion, and positive emotion, among them the insula and medial prefrontal cortex. These regions grow in size and power with increased practice. The insula is an empathy center of the brain, so we effectively become better at empathy, while the medial prefrontal region is associated with compassion, positive emotion, happiness, and joy.

Loving-kindness is also associated with spiritual states of consciousness, which means that as we develop it through meditative practice, it becomes easier to access these states.

Cultivating Compassion

Researchers at the Max Planck Institute for Human Cognitive and Brain Sciences in Leipzig, Germany, together with Matthieu Ricard, a Buddhist monk and scientist, suggested that emotional exhaustion, a form of burnout, is a type of empathy fatigue. To test this, they split 60 volunteers into two groups, half of whom practiced loving-kindness for a week while the other half focused on cultivating feelings of empathy for others.[5]

At the end of the trial, the volunteers were shown videos of people suffering. Those who had practiced empathy resonated with the suffering they saw, but they also experienced stress and negative emotions, as if they were emotionally overwhelmed and unable to extract themselves from that suffering.

The researchers then invited those individuals to practice loving-kindness, which focused on cultivating love and compassion. The volunteers' negative emotions subsequently disappeared, and they were able to develop empathy and compassion without feeling emotionally overwhelmed.

One of the reasons for this type of effect, says Kristen Neff, an associate professor of educational psychology at the University of Texas at Austin, USA, is that empathy is 'I feel *with* you,' while compassion is 'I feel *for* you.' When we feel compassion, we share the person's suffering, as with empathy, but we also have an honest desire to see the person become free of their suffering. Some of our attention shifts from sympathizing with their pain to wishing them freedom from it. This is what loving-kindness practice helps us to do.

The Health Benefits of Meditation

The reported cognitive and psychological benefits of meditation and mindfulness practice are numerous, and what follows is merely a small sample of some of the research findings. As there are a vast number of meditation studies, I've summarized reviews and meta-analyses (large combined statistical analyses of many individual studies) of randomized controlled trials.

Many of the benefits of mindfulness stem from the fact that the practice helps us observe our thoughts without engaging with them. It reduces stress and anxiety because we're able to notice the patterns of thinking or beliefs that give rise to stress, or to observe a stressful feeling without being sucked into it. The net effects can be numerous.

> *Meditation studies show reductions in stress and anxiety and increases in self-esteem as we learn to notice our thoughts and beliefs in a less judgmental way.*

In 2013, researchers at the University of Montreal in Canada conducted a review of more than 200 studies involving over 12,000 people and showed that mindfulness meditation is 'an effective treatment for a variety of psychological disorders,' but that it was especially effective for reducing depression, anxiety, and stress.[6]

Similarly, Johns Hopkins University researchers in the USA published a systematic review and meta-analysis in 2014 of 47 trials involving 3,515 participants and concluded that meditation practice resulted in significant reductions in anxiety, depression, and pain.[7] They also suggested that clinicians should include meditation practices as part of a wider treatment plan for optimizing mental health.

Meditation has also been shown to help reduce the chances of relapse in people with substance abuse issues. According to researchers at the University of Utah in the USA, the practice helps those with addictive behavior to become aware of the urge without giving in to it. It can also alter brain receptors associated with drug and alcohol use, even helping to alter the way pleasure is processed.[8]

Meditation can help improve learning and memory, as a Harvard study showed. Researchers used MRI to compare the brains of participants practicing meditation over eight weeks (who had never tried meditation before the study) with participants who weren't doing the practice. At the end of the program, the meditators had an increase in gray matter in brain regions associated with learning and memory.[9]

And meditation can be used in pain management, too. In 2020, a meta-analysis of 60 randomized controlled trials involving over 6,000 participants published by researchers at the University of Utah showed that meditation and other mind–body therapies (for example, hypnosis, guided imagery, and cognitive behavioral therapy) reduced acute pain, chronic pain, and also post-surgical pain.[10]

It also helped reduce reliance on opioid drugs for pain management. The effects on pain can be attributed to the fact that meditation trains us to observe pain without being drawn into the experience of it quite as much.

Slowing the Aging Process

There are some surprising physiological benefits to meditation and mindfulness practice, too, one of which is that it appears to slow aging. It's not entirely clear how, but it may be that by reducing stress, meditation helps many systems of the body, including the immune system and processes involved in cellular repair, to work more optimally.

One of the measured effects of meditation is that it can reduce inflammation, which plays a significant role in aging. So much so, in fact, that aging researchers now refer to it as 'inflammaging,' a term first coined by Claudio Franceschi, Emeritus Professor in the Department of Experimental Pathology at Italy's University of Bologna.[11]

A 2016 Carnegie Mellon University randomized controlled trial involving 35 stressed job-seeking adults examined the effect of mindfulness practice on inflammation, specifically on an inflammatory biomarker called Interleukin-6, which is an indicator of systemic inflammation and inflammatory disease risk and is also implicated in aging.[12]

Around half of the volunteers participated in an intensive three-day mindfulness meditation retreat, and the rest attended a three-day relaxation retreat without the mindfulness component. Brain scans were taken before the trial and after three days, and blood samples were taken before and at a four-month follow-up.

Mindfulness practice caused a significant reduction in Interleukin-6 levels. The brain scans showed that, unlike the relaxation training, mindfulness meditation had increased the number of connections in brain regions associated with attention and self-control, and had coupled brain regions that helped with self-control and concentration and were involved in resilience to stress. Using statistical analysis, the researchers further showed that these brain changes were associated with much of the reduction in inflammation.

Over a six-week period in 2008, Harvard University researchers compared people practicing meditation with those who did none. Analyzing blood samples from the participants, they found that meditation impacted more than 1,500 genes in novice meditators and more than 2,200 genes in experienced meditators.

In the novices, almost 900 genes were turned up and almost 600 were turned down. Examining some of the affected genes, lead researcher Dr. Herbert Benson noted that meditation seemed to be slowing aging at a cellular level.[13]

The Role of Telomeres

Researchers at the universities of California at Davis, San Francisco, and Irvine studying volunteers who attended an intensive meditation retreat over a longer period of three months found that they even had higher levels of an important enzyme known as telomerase in their cells.[14] Telomerase helps build our telomeres – the aging beacons of our DNA.

> **Essentially, intensive meditation practice slows the rate of aging at a genetic level.**

The kindfulness practice we explored earlier – in which the focus of the meditation is building a sentiment of kindness, love, and compassion – seems to have an even more profound effect on telomeres. In 2018, psychologist Barbara Fredrickson and her team at the University of North Carolina at Chapel Hill in the USA studied telomere length in volunteers who practiced either loving-kindness or mindfulness daily for six weeks, or who did no meditation practice.[15] Telomere length was measured at the beginning and end of the period.

Telomere length is considered one of the most accurate indicators of a person's biological age, and longer telomeres are indicative of a lower biological age. Essentially, we have two ages: our chronological age, which is the number of years we've been alive, and our biological age, which is the effective age of our body.

There's often a disparity between the two in that people who follow a healthy lifestyle often have a biological age that's less than their chronological age, and those who have an unhealthy lifestyle typically tend to have a biological age that's more than their chronological age.

Fredrickson's study showed that telomere length slowed a little in those volunteers who did the mindfulness practice, although not much. Perhaps a noticeable protection of telomeres requires a more sustained or intense practice of mindfulness, as suggested by the aforementioned study that measured telomere length after a three-month meditation retreat. However, in the group who practiced loving-kindness, there was *no* noticeable telomere shortening during the six-week period.

While the underlying mechanism for the seemingly protective effect of loving-kindness practice on telomeres isn't yet fully clear, it appears likely that an anti-inflammatory effect plays a role.

The Nerve of Compassion

Loving-kindness (*metta*) has also been shown to increase activity of the vagus nerve (a nerve that plays a key role in the parasympathetic – rest-and-digest – nervous system). This leads to an increase in heart rate variability (HRV) – the beat-to-beat variation in heart rate that's mediated by the vagus nerve and is also known as vagal tone. Loving-kindness practice has been shown to increase vagal tone.

The vagus nerve also plays a key anti-inflammatory role in the body through the inflammatory reflex, which was first identified by Kevin J. Tracey, Professor of Neurosurgery at The Feinstein Institutes for Medical Research in the USA.[16] Here, the vagus nerve senses when there's enough inflammation for healing to occur and signals a turning down of the TNF-alpha gene, effectively halting further inflammation.

Studies have shown that people practicing loving-kindness for several weeks tend to have not only increased vagal tone but also a lower inflammatory response to stress. In a 2018 meta-analysis, scientists found that people with stage 4 cancer who had high vagal tone lived much longer than those with low vagal tone.[17] The researchers pointed to the likely anti-inflammatory effect of high vagal tone at a time when the patients' drug treatments were no longer providing benefit as the most likely reason for their extra years.

You may wonder why kindfulness practices should increase vagal tone in the first place. The answer lies in our evolution. Human babies are born prematurely in comparison with the offspring of many other animal species; puppies, for example, are walking within a few days of birth, yet human babies need around nine months to master the same feat. As a result, human babies need parental care for many months (and years) before they're able to fend for themselves.

Over eons of evolution, a close relationship formed between our feelings of care and compassion for our young as we reared them and the activity of our autonomic nervous system (ANS), in particular the vagus nerve.

Feelings of care and compassion essentially became associated with vagus nerve activity. For this reason, the vagus nerve is often called the caretaking nerve or even the nerve of compassion. This understanding was first put forward by Stephen Porges, Distinguished University Scientist at the University of Indiana and Professor of Psychiatry at the University of North Carolina at Chapel Hill, and is encapsulated in polyvagal theory.

In effect, these days, feelings of compassion increase vagus nerve activity, increasing HRV and vagal tone, and also produce an anti-inflammatory effect. It may be that the anti-inflammatory effect induced by loving-kindness practice was also responsible for the protection of telomeres in Barbara Fredrickson's six-week study.

The Power of the Breath

The slower loss of telomeres in those who practice loving-kindness might also be down to slower meditative breathing. Just like those who practice other forms of repetitive prayer, people who practice loving-kindness tend to repeat the phrases slowly on the out breath. This has the effect of slowing breathing, but also of breathing less and taking in less oxygen.

While this may sound dangerous, the opposite is true: for short periods, it can be hugely beneficial. The effect is a slight increase in blood carbon dioxide levels, which ultimately causes the body to make more efficient use of oxygen. Slow breathing practices have helped athletes outperform their previous records, and studies have suggested that breathing less can actually increase lifespan.[18]

> *Along with slow breathing practices, faster meditative breathing, performed in a controlled way, can also have significant benefits.*

Tummo, also known as fire breath, is an ancient Tibetan breathing practice that involves visualizing the body as a large, hollow, inflated balloon with a small ball of fire and warmth burning within, followed by alternating fast and deep breathing with periods of controlled breath-holding. It was developed to enable practitioners to generate body heat in icy caves.

Advanced Buddhist practitioners of Tummo have demonstrated its effects by sitting high up a mountain in subzero temperatures wearing only a wet sheet that had been immersed in ice water. The sheet quickly dried, due to the large amount of heat generated in the body by the breath practice.

The Wim Hof Method

The Tummo breathing technique has been adapted in the West by the Dutch extreme athlete Wim Hof – nicknamed The Iceman – whose Wim Hof Method is based on breathing, cold therapy, and commitment. Hof has held multiple world records for enduring extreme cold, including swimming under ice for almost 197 feet (60 meters), running a half marathon barefoot over ice and snow, and sitting with his whole body in direct contact with ice for almost two hours, all without enduring any burns to his skin.

In a study at Radboud University Medical Center in the Netherlands, Hof was injected with an E. coli endotoxin – a safe way of provoking a bacterial immune response without infecting volunteers with the live bacteria. Typically, on injection, the immune system responds with a high production of pro-inflammatory cytokines, as well as flu-like symptoms of fever, chills, and headache. However, when Hof was injected, he produced 50 percent less of these cytokines and produced a large anti-inflammatory response. He also exhibited very few flu-like symptoms.[19]

In a later study, Hof trained 12 volunteers in his meditation and breathing methods, each of whom were subsequently injected with the bacterial endotoxin. Their immune responses were compared with those of 12 people who didn't undergo the training. In a similar way to Hof himself, his trainees showed a significant dampening of the pro-inflammatory response to the endotoxin, when compared with the control group, and also showed far fewer flu-type symptoms.[20]

Meditation as a Spiritual Practice

Meditation has been practiced for thousands of years, long before the advent of brain scanners or blood sampling. Many people pursue meditation as a spiritual practice. They don't meditate because it changes their brain, makes them more positive, boosts their immune system, or helps them live longer – they do it because it helps them experience deeper self-awareness and an intuitive sense of life and existence.

It's commonly believed that the purpose of meditation is to help us stop thinking, and as a result many people give up the practice after a couple of weeks because they find themselves still thinking thoughts during a 10-minute sitting. While the mind does indeed tend to become more still during meditation, that isn't the goal of those who pursue it as a spiritual practice.

> *The practice in meditation isn't not to think, but to notice that you're thinking. The goal is awareness; stillness is a side effect.*

Advanced practitioners of meditation say that we illuminate our thinking with our awareness and then rest in that awareness. With awareness, we can be in a silent place or in an extremely noisy one, but no matter where we are and in what context, we can still feel calm and still. The setting in which we find ourselves becomes part of the practice – filled with objects, noises, and experiences on which we can let our awareness settle.

As the practice deepens, we become more aware of our own being – the spiritual presence deep within ourselves that gives rise to thoughts and feelings. The goal of advanced meditation practice is to bathe in this awareness. In time, we learn to spend more and more of our time in that mental and emotional space of awareness – not only during a meditation session, but also in everyday life as we go about our business. Routine tasks then become part of the meditation practice, and life itself becomes a meditation.

Meditation is ultimately a spiritual practice, then, but even with just a little practice, its fruits can help us experience more peace and joy in our lives.

Living in the Present Moment

Advanced practitioners of meditation also notice that objects and the environment take on a deeper, richer appearance. Colors seem to be more vibrant, objects more real. This is a perception shift and it occurs as a consequence of having more of our awareness on the present moment instead of ruminating about the past, worrying about the future, or planning our next step in life.

Meditation trains us to focus on now. And in the now, we begin to notice more of it – the things that surround us, colors, textures, and even the happenings in the lives of loved ones that we sometimes miss when we're preoccupied with the contents of our own mind.

So, if you choose to practice meditation, instead of trying to have no thoughts, try instead to have awareness. Then, whatever you're aware *of* – whether its thoughts, sensations, sounds, objects, or circumstances – will become part of a constant practice of meditation. Advanced practitioners teach that we should bathe in awareness and that it will set us free from our mental and emotional suffering.

If you're looking for instruction on meditation, there are many good books on the subject. I recommend *Wherever You Go, There You Are* by Jon Kabat-Zinn, who is Executive Director of the Center for Mindfulness in Medicine at the University of Massachusetts Medical School; *How to Meditate*, by American Tibetan Buddhist Pema Chödrön; and *Mindfulness in Plain English*, by Sri Lankan Theravada Buddhist monk Bhante Gunaratana.

CHAPTER 3

Trapped and Released Emotion

I was walking by a river with my dog, Oscar, one day when he spotted a group of swans. *This is new*, he must have thought – he was quite young at the time and hadn't yet encountered these creatures – and as he did with every dog or person he ever saw, he went over to say 'hello.'

As he approached the swans, one stretched its wings wide open, made a loud rasping sound, and moved toward him. Oscar took fright and ran back to me with a wee yelp. Once safely by my side, he shook himself vigorously, as if he'd just emerged wet from the river and was drying himself, then urinated on a tree before running off to play with his ball. It was as if nothing had happened.

We could learn a lot from animals if we paid them enough attention, although I'm not suggesting you should urinate on a tree or anything like that when someone's mean to you. *Shaking it off* is an instinct that some animals have which allows them to release the effects of stress, fear, or some other negative emotion from their nervous system, and something similar works for humans too.

Movement, exercise, dance, yoga, or even a dog-style shake can all help to relieve some of the pent-up emotions that many of us accumulate on an almost daily basis. But why is it that negative emotions build up in the body in the first place?

A Two-Way Street

Science has shown that the mind affects the body and the body affects the mind. Emotional tension usually creates physical tension in the neck and shoulders. Some people grind their teeth, while others suffer from tension headaches as the muscles above and behind the eyes contract. A tired mind is often mirrored in a tired body. Chronic stress, overwhelm, or even depression can leave a person feeling physically exhausted.

Fear causes hairs on the back of the neck to rise. A blush usually follows a feeling of self-consciousness, embarrassment, or shame. Sexual excitement produces an erection in males and erect nipples in females. We also smile when we feel happy; we don't have to remember to smile – it happens spontaneously. Similarly, we don't have to remember to scrunch up our face or tense our jaw and shoulders when we feel stressed; these things happen by themselves. The body is a mirror of our mental and emotional states.

We're all familiar with these physical effects of emotion because they're so commonplace, and they tell us that our feelings aren't *just* in our mind. Prolonged stress can build up in the body. It's first noticeable in the muscles – most obviously those on the face, but it also lodges in the upper body, often leaving us with 'knots' in our shoulders and a sore neck.

This is why massage feels so good – releasing the tension from the muscles often simultaneously releases it from the mind, from that which *causes* the physical tension. Sometimes a massage will release a little bit of tension, enough to ease us into a relaxed and soothed state; other times, if the therapist prods deeply enough, despite the physical pain, the release can feel nothing short of sublime. And there are times when it can produce such a large emotional release that it leaves the recipient in tears.

This two-way street, in which the mind affects the body and vice versa, is why tensing the jaw and shoulders or making jerky movements aren't just things you do when you feel stressed – in themselves, they can actually *make* you feel stressed. It's why 'shaking it off' can help to remove pent-up emotions that aren't lodged too deeply. And it's also why engaging in vigorous exercise at the end of the working day can go some way to relieving much of the stress we've accumulated in our muscles.

An Accumulation of Stress

Why is it that the body seems to be in sync with our emotional states? Long before our early ancestors developed language, they communicated their feelings through facial expressions, body language, and physical gestures. Happy states were communicated with bright eyes and a smile, sadness with a frown, and anger through raised vocalizations and aggressive physical posturing.

Anthropologists tell us that these expressions are consistent across all cultures – even those that have been isolated from civilization until recently – which has convinced them that they're innate. Over eons, emotional states simply became correlated with their physical expression, so that today, each emotion has a physical counterpart.

> *Emotions leave 'charges' in our muscles and our nervous system as we tense our body in response to mental and emotional stress.*

Over time, these emotional charges can add up. Repeated stress not only accumulates in our muscles, it also builds up in the nervous system. Stress stimulates the sympathetic nervous system – the fight-or-flight portion of the autonomic nervous system (ANS). ANS activity increases when we're under stress and decreases when we feel calm, and it's not designed to be in a heightened state for long periods of time.

Many of us push our pain and negative emotions deep inside our body, as if we're stuffing old clothes into a box and closing the lid. However, while we've all experienced the temporary sense of calm this can bring, the more we contain our negative emotions in this way, the less likely they are to remain hidden from view. Eventually, when our buttons are pressed, they'll explode out of us in a blaze of anger or tears.

This can happen at seemingly random moments, or in response to a particular person's words or behavior, or even when a sound or a situation reminds us (or reminds the body) of a past traumatic experience. There can be serious physical effects to bottling up our pain and negative emotions, especially if we never release them.

The Role of Personality in Disease

The idea that there could be a link between mental and emotional states and disease was once considered pseudoscience. In 1985, an editorial in *The New England Journal of Medicine* made the mainstream position at the time quite clear – this supposed connection was, it said, 'largely folklore.'

However, in the years since, sufficient evidence has accumulated to turn that position completely on its head. In his book *When the Body Says No*, Gabor Maté, physician and internationally renowned expert on trauma, addiction, and child development, remarks that 'such dismissals are no longer tenable.'

Research now shows a clear connection between some aspects of personality and a person's susceptibility to specific diseases. For example, studies have revealed a link between the Type C personality and the thickness and prevalence of some cancerous tumors. The Type C personality is described as 'cooperative, unassertive, passive, patient, and suppresses negative emotion.' Type C individuals tend to repress negative emotions, especially anger, but at the same time, they often try hard to maintain an outward appearance of happiness. So strong is this connection that in her research, Lydia Temoshok, former Professor of Medicine at the University of Maryland in the USA, referred to Type C personality as 'cancer prone.'[1]

Some research has shown links between the Type C personality and some cancers, including breast cancer. For example, a 1991 study that assessed the personality traits of more than 600 people with cancer of the colon or rectum found that, when compared with a matched control group, they showed 'elements of denial and the repression of anger and other negative emotions.'[2]

And a large Johns Hopkins University study that began in the 1940s and ran for around 40 years reported that 'cancer patients tend to deny and repress conflictual impulses and emotions to a higher degree than do other people.'[3]

Before we go any further, let me make it clear that such research findings do not imply that repressed emotion *causes* cancer, only that there's a correlation between them. Negative emotions don't cause cancer, but people of the same personality type often have similar coping styles, and some styles generate higher levels of physiological stress than others.

This in itself doesn't cause disease, but it can increase the risk by upsetting the immune system and the body's natural homeostatic balance. When combined with a person's genetic predisposition and some other environmental factors, a cancer recipe can more readily brew in a Type C personality body.

Other personality types are connected to different conditions. In one of her studies, Temoshok compared personality traits among patients who had malignant melanoma, cardiovascular disease, and a control group with no medical conditions.[4] She found that the malignant melanoma patients tended to deny being upset or anxious and were more likely to suppress negative emotions (Type C).

On the other hand, cardiovascular disease patients were more likely to be Type A personality; while Type C people suppress anger, Type A people much more freely express it, but to the extent that they have a particular attitude and a tendency to be outwardly aggressive.

Anger, Hostility, and the Heart

Research has now also strongly linked anger, hostility, and aggression with coronary artery disease. In fact, a doctor can sometimes obtain as much information about a person's risk of cardiovascular disease from a short personality questionnaire as they can from one that asks about diet and lifestyle habits.

From the 1950s, research began to show that Type A personality males (aggressive, hostile, excessively driven, competitive, time conscious, dominant) had higher incidences of cardiovascular disease than other personality types. More recent research has shown that it's the anger and hostility component of the personality that's related to coronary artery health, not the personality type itself.[5]

Hostility is generally thought of as expressed contempt or an aggressive attitude. It's composed of three parts: cognitive, affective, and behavioral. The cognitive (mental) part is that hostile people typically have negative beliefs about, and cynical attitudes toward, others, particularly around the idea that others are motivated by their own selfish concerns. Hostile people also tend to be mistrusting of others and even paranoid. The affective part can be broad, ranging from anger to rage, and hostile people are usually irritable and resentful.

Hostility tends to be expressed verbally or physically, either with aggression or passive-aggression. Verbal aggression is the most common form and is often done spitefully, hatefully, resentfully, with sarcasm, or argumentatively, with the person taking an opposing stance seemingly for the sake of it. In other words, it starts with the beliefs and attitude, which produce a feeling that's expressed as an angry outburst, often with verbal or physical aggression.

While all this paints an apparently negative picture of hostile people, I think that most of us, in certain moments in our lives, have shown hostility – in our responses to particular people, say, or to particular circumstances. Feeling angry or hostile from time to time will do little or no harm; it's being consistently hostile over long spans of time that can be damaging.

Consistent hostility usually betrays some underlying hurt. It's been said that the people who are the most aggressive are often the most hurt or afraid, and that those who act the strongest are often the ones who feel (or who have felt) the weakest.

The Roots of Hostility

Although it's not always the case, hostility tends to begin in childhood, when it can be learned from parents.[6] A hostile parent and an unhappy childhood are strong predictors of hostility in adulthood. Hostility can also be the result of parental behavior or treatment; it can derive from an unavailable parent with high job involvement who had little time for a child, or even be due to abuse or neglect.

Bullying by a sibling can also provoke hostility that's rooted in defensiveness and it can carry over into adulthood. While these trends aren't absolute, they generally indicate that the seeds of hostility are often sown in childhood.

Consistent hostility can have severe health consequences for the heart. In the UK, a University College London review of 25 published studies found that anger and hostility were associated with poorer prognosis in people who already have coronary heart disease, but also increased coronary heart disease episodes in a healthy population. Left unchecked, hostility can be fatal.[7]

There are some differences between men and women in this regard, though. In studies of healthy people, the association between anger, hostility, and heart disease seems to be stronger in men than it is in women.

Some of the research has explored hostility in relationships. Observations of couples interacting for short periods of time show that individuals who are more hostile or aggressive tend to have higher levels of calcification in their arteries. In the same studies, people who tend to be kind, gentle, and affectionate tend to have healthier arteries – relatively speaking.[8]

It's almost as if, if we harden our emotional heart toward others, so we harden in our physical heart. Emotional hardening seems to be mirrored in the cardiovascular system.

Adverse Childhood Experiences

In 1995, the US Centers for Disease Control and Protection and the Kaiser Permanente healthcare organization in California, USA, coined the term Adverse Childhood Experiences, or ACE, to refer to the different types of adversity that children can experience in their home environment.

Adverse Childhood Experiences are much more common than most of us might imagine. More than two thirds of the US population has experienced at least one ACE and almost a quarter has experienced three or more. ACEs can include various forms of physical or mental abuse, neglect, household dysfunction, living with a parent who has a mental illnesses or is suicidal, witnessing domestic violence, chronic poverty, experiences with racism, or even violence in the community.

ACEs can cause toxic stress, a term coined by the US National Scientific Council on the Developing Child to describe the excessive activation of the stress response systems in the body on account of trauma. Toxic stress can have severe detrimental effects on a developing child's brain, immune system, and cardiovascular system, and even how it experiences pain.[9]

If a growing child doesn't have supportive adult relationships to help buffer toxic stress, research shows that it can lead to depression, anxiety, chronic pain, arthritis, fibromyalgia, cardiovascular disease, and autoimmune disease in adulthood. Child abuse in particular is associated with increases in rates of cancer, cardiovascular disease, and diabetes, as well as multiple mental health conditions.

Researchers assign an ACE score to indicate the number of different categories of ACE a child experiences. The higher the ACE score in childhood, the more likely the individual is to suffer chronic mental or physical conditions in adulthood.

ACEs and Depression

In a study that related childhood ACE score to depression in adulthood, for example, the rate of chronic depression in those with a score of four or more was more than five times higher in women and about three times higher in men than it was in people with an ACE score of zero.[10]

Some recent research suggests that this increased risk of depression might be related to epigenetic changes that occur on account of the trauma – these are small chemical changes to a gene that affect the way it functions. Researchers at Yale University and the Child Mind Institute in New York in the USA identified epigenetic changes in a group of 94 children who had suffered trauma, compared with 96 children who hadn't. They found a link between the trauma and specific epigenetic changes in three important genes that related to an increased risk of depression.[11]

Health services around the world spend billions on antidepressant drugs, yet for a great number of people these are, in effect, treating painful events that took place years, even decades, earlier. The drugs treat the brain chemistry associated with the way a person feels *now*, but not the underlying trauma that produced it.

According to psychiatrist, author, and trauma expert Bessel van der Kolk, in his book *The Body Keeps the Score*, this may be why antidepressants tend to be less effective in people with a history of sexual abuse or trauma.

People with an ACE score of four or more are also 40–60 percent more likely to be physically inactive or severely obese in adulthood than those with no ACEs.[12] They are also two to four times more likely to smoke and be in poor health and have a four- to twelvefold increase in substance abuse, alcoholism, depression, and suicide attempt.

ACEs and the Immune System

Many adults who suffered abuse as a child are hypervigilant: constantly on alert, they scan their surroundings for potential threats and instinctively check for an exit in every room or building they enter, as if to register an escape route should the need arise. They immediately notice people's scars and tattoos and subconsciously equate them with risk. They're also generally hypersensitive to facial expressions that convey mistrust or any form of aggression, and can struggle to tell the difference between safety and danger.

But this hypersensitivity and hypervigilance can be mirrored in the immune system too, where the person is far more at risk of developing allergies or autoimmune conditions than someone without an ACE history.

In *The Body Keeps the Score*, van der Kolk shares an example of a study that he and colleagues at Massachusetts General Hospital undertook that involved 24 women, half of whom had been traumatized by parental sexual abuse.[13] They found that the women who had been abused had abnormalities in the ratio between important immune system memory cells; this ratio indicated that their immune systems were abnormally vigilant to threats, not unlike the women themselves.

Many other researchers now share this view of a link between childhood trauma and immune dysfunction in adulthood. People with higher ACE scores are much more likely to be hospitalized for an autoimmune disease, even decades into their adult years. In particular, one study found a 100 percent increased risk of rheumatoid arthritis in adults who had had an ACE score greater than two as children.[14] ACE score is also linked with chronic pain in adulthood and research suggests that it's caused by disruption in the development of pain-processing regions of the brain.[15]

The Impact of Neglect

The human body has evolved to be able to distinguish playful or compassionate touch, like that of motherly love, from aggressive contact. The body knows the difference. Playful or compassionate touch is indicative of a healthy environment and is rewarded with optimum growth of the brain and body and the activation of systems that help maintain and heal it. Aggressive touch, on the other hand, indicates danger and stimulates stress control systems.

The gentle touch of motherly love plays a crucial role in the development of the touch and pain-sensing 'nociceptive pathways' in the brain of an infant. It ensures that they receive the activation and nutrients they need for optimum growth; however, the development of the pathways can be stunted if a child is neglected, rendering it more sensitive to touch and pain.

In a double punch, neglected or abused children are more likely to experience physical health problems as adults, and they also suffer more pain because of them. Indeed, in a study of more than 18,000 people across 10 countries, the neglect, abuse, family violence, or criminal behavior they experienced in childhood was strongly associated with pain in adulthood from chronic physical conditions.[16]

One of the most striking effects in children who are abused or neglected is smaller physical size: the bones grow more slowly, the head circumference is smaller, and even the heart is smaller. This is the result of reduced activity of growth hormone genes and reduced production of oxytocin, the kindness hormone, which plays an important role in the construction of heart muscle cells as well as many other cell types in the body.

Brain development is also stunted. The orbitofrontal cortex, which sits behind the orbits of the eyes, doesn't develop according to a preset genetic program but builds almost entirely in response to a child's environment.

The Bucharest Early Intervention Project, a large study that tracked the physical and neurological growth and development of thousands of children who were raised in Romanian orphanages, together with related research from orphanages and other institutions around the globe, has shown us that the brains of children who are institutionalized at a young age and aren't loved and cared for, or lovingly parented, and where no one is responsive to their needs, develop 'holes' in the orbitofrontal cortex.[17] The holes are regions where growth is much less than it should be.

In a sense, a child's emotional environment provides the soil and nutrients that the orbitofrontal cortex needs for growth. When a child doesn't receive enough love, and experiences much less positive emotion than they typically would while growing up, the soil is depleted, and the nourishment needed by the orbitofrontal cortex is denied; as a result, its growth falters.

On the upside, research shows that if such children are fostered or adopted into good family environments – particularly before the age of two, while the orbitofrontal cortex is still developing – much of the previously stunted neurological and physical growth returns to normal.[18] As the emotions are fed the nourishment of love, so the body follows suit, and its growth reflects the changes in the psyche.

Releasing Trauma and Suppressed Emotion

When University of Texas professor James Pennebaker asked students to write about the thoughts and feelings that arose from their painful, stressful, or traumatic life experiences, whether from childhood or adulthood, for 20 minutes on four consecutive days, he noted that the exercise led to improvements in their mental and physical health.

Expressive writing, as Pennebaker later called this technique, served as a release value that eased some of the students' emotional stress and the underlying toxic stress that it caused.

In one study, Pennebaker recorded visits to the student medical center over the course of a few months as an indicator of general health. He found that the individuals who had written about traumatic events visited the center much less often than those who, as a comparison, had been asked to write about their more trivial life experiences.

In another study, he invited volunteers to speak about their traumatic experiences on a tape recorder instead of writing them down. This time, he measured muscle tension, hand temperature, heart rate, and blood pressure, all of which are indicators of stress or arousal. When the volunteers began to speak about their traumatic experiences, their stress and arousal levels increased, as would be expected when aspects of a trauma are recalled. But as they continued speaking, these stress and arousal levels dropped significantly, to way below what they had been before the study began.

Even six weeks after the study, the volunteers' blood pressure remained lower than it had been before they'd uttered the first word into the tape recorder. Pennebaker's research shows that remembering painful things can be painful, but once they're spoken about or written down, they lose some of their grip on us.[19]

Words that Heal

In his book *Expressive Writing*, Pennebaker describes a study in which volunteers who wrote expressively of their traumatic experiences were also found to have improved immune function.[20] After just four 20-minute writing sessions, they had greater T-cell activity, as well as elevations in other immune markers in their blood. And these levels were still raised six weeks after the study.

Once some of the trauma had been released, its suppressing effects on the immune system were effectively removed. Thus, when there's less toxic stress on it, the immune system can be more responsive to everyday opportunistic infections.

In another study, Pennebaker found that the immune responses of most individuals to a toxin was significantly higher after they had completed an exercise to release pent-up negative emotion that was associated with hurt or trauma.

The expressive writing exercise that Pennebaker pioneered is straightforward. We simply write about a hurtful, traumatic, or stressful event for about 20 minutes on four consecutive days. The professor's guidelines recommend first stating the issue and then writing down what happened, how it felt then, how it feels now, and how it's impacted our life. As they move from the first to the fourth day of writing, many people find they eventually start writing more positively about their experiences – about what they've learned from them.

In one of Pennebaker's studies, volunteers who had experienced sexual trauma as children, and who had a history of health problems in adulthood, showed an incredible 50 percent reduction in hospital visits after doing the four-day practice.

Developing Self-Awareness

One of the consequences of Pennebaker's technique is that it can help a person become more self-aware – to know themselves better, their feelings and needs, who they are, and what makes them tick.

From a neuroscience perspective, self-awareness seems to play an important role in the release of painful emotions because it helps to link frontal regions of the brain that are associated with higher brain functions – such as concentration, decision-making, and the experience of positive emotions – with the amygdala, which processes fear and anxiety and is involved in the processing of most of our emotional pain.

Most frontal regions of the brain don't directly connect with the amygdala, and this is why positive thinking, although immensely beneficial for many aspects of life, doesn't always help when we're dealing with trauma or negative emotions that are extremely painful and buried more deeply.

However, with added self-awareness, the frontal regions link with regions associated with sensing the internal state of the body, which in turn link with the amygdala. It's this multiple connectivity that helps us to access the emotional brain from a more conscious adult perspective, instead of a reactionary one. In order to manage ourselves better, therefore, it helps to get to know ourselves better.

Knowing ourselves can mean acknowledging our pain instead of burying it, making friends with ourselves and how we feel, and learning that it's okay not to feel okay.

Writing helps us to get stuff out of our system, but that's not the only thing that's important here: writing also helps us to become more aware of how we're really *feeling* about things. There's a balance to be struck. On the one hand, focusing on the positives is great for helping us to feel more positive, but there are times when that's not possible – times when pain or trauma have neared the surface and have to be dealt with in another way. While some degree of pain can be transmuted by a more positive focus, that which is more deeply held needs a greater level of self-awareness and an exploration of our feelings.

Conscious Breathing Practices

Breathing and movement practices such as meditation and yoga can also help to release painful emotions because they calm stress or anxiety through conscious control of the breath. Breathing is usually unconscious, but it's one of the autonomic (unconscious) functions of the body that we *can* control.

Through conscious breath control practices, including the Tummo and Wim Hof methods we discussed in the previous chapter, we can in effect 'hack into' the autonomic nervous system (ANS). Breathing slowly, for example, relaxes us into a greater parasympathetic state and at the same time reduces sympathetic activity. In fact, some breathing exercises can go a long way to removing the effects of toxic stress.

Much of the ANS-hacking effect is mediated by the vagus nerve. It connects the brain and our internal organs, but only 20 percent of its fibers run from the brain to the body. About 80 percent run the other way, from the body to the brain. This is why breath and movement exercises are so helpful when we need to calm ourselves and release stress.

No matter what may have happened to us in our past, conscious breathing practices can give us hope.

> **Breathing practices help us tap directly into important physiological processes, boosting those that are good for us and reducing those that are linked with stress.**

However, if breathing practices are used as part of a strategy for dealing with buried negative emotion, they're best supplemented with self-awareness practices such as expressive writing, or working with a trained therapist.

Breathing and movement practices are excellent for calming emotional charges in the moment, and even gradually in the longer term, but they can be especially powerful when coupled with techniques that can help us befriend ourselves. A good resource for breathing exercises is the book *Breath* by James Nestor.

Energy work – EFT and EMDR

Emotional Freedom Technique (EFT) is another method that can help us release trauma. It involves tapping on a series of acupuncture points on the body while acknowledging a pain or trauma and making repetitive statements around self-acceptance.

In 2016, I traveled to Australia's Gold Coast to speak at a conference called Mind Heart Connect: Creating Resilient Lives, which was organized jointly by Dr. Peta Stapleton, Professor of Clinical Psychology at Bond University, and social entrepreneur Kate Helder. During my time there I learned EFT from one of the speakers, Dr. Lori Leyden, a psychotherapist and specialist in trauma healing.

Lori has traveled around the world for decades working with survivors of trauma. Largely using The Grace Process, a seven-step spiritual and somatic formula she developed that includes EFT, she has helped thousands of orphaned survivors of the 1994 Rwandan genocide to process and heal the trauma of witnessing the slaughter of their family members and other villagers, as well as vicious attacks on themselves. She has also helped survivors of US school shootings come to terms with what they witnessed and to release toxic stress from their mind and body.

EFT is often considered pseudoscience, and yet studies show it has helped thousands of survivors of sexual abuse, people dealing with anxiety, and many war veterans to recover from post-traumatic stress disorder (PTSD).[21] The technique is starting to emerge into the mainstream, an advance that has been helped by MRI scans that show its neurological effects.

In a 2019 study of people with food cravings, Dr. Peta Stapleton showed that daily EFT practice by overweight adults eliminated their cravings; and not only that: MRI scans revealed physical changes in key brain regions associated with cravings.[22]

Eye movement desensitization and reprocessing (EMDR), a psychotherapy technique developed in 1988 by American psychologist Francine Shapiro, has also been extremely successful in helping people alleviate the distress associated with traumatic memories and other adverse life events.

As we'll explore in the next chapter, early humans lived in relative peace and calm (when compared with the frenetic pace of modern life). As most of their time was spent outside, surveying the African savanna for food and signs of danger, it was natural for them to make rapid left and right eye movements as they did so. These eye movements thus became connected with parasympathetic activity over vast expanses of time.

The basis of EMDR is that therapist-directed conscious left and right eye movements hack into this ancient correlation and allow us to access, and boost, relaxing parasympathetic activity. If this is done while recalling a traumatic experience, it helps the brain connect it with positive feelings instead of negative ones.

EMDR has helped reduce symptoms of PTSD in thousands of soldiers returning from Iraq and Afghanistan, and since 2020, it's been listed by the American Psychological Association as an evidence-based treatment for this condition.

CHAPTER 4

Nature

Over millions of years of evolution, we humans have spent 99.99 percent of our time in natural surroundings, and just 0.01 percent in a built-up environment. Modern genetic analysis suggests our species, *Homo sapiens*, branched off from other species around 260,000 years ago. They lived out their lives in Africa's tropical savanna (grasslands), having migrated from the lush landscape known as the Makgadikgadi-Okavango wetland in what is today Botswana. Modern humans emerged from there and migrated to Europe, Asia, and Australia in several waves more than 100,000 years ago.[1]

While stress is common in human populations today, our early cousins, if they had possessed complex language, wouldn't have coined a word for it because they experienced it so rarely. Other than the natural stressors of hunger and the occasional scrap, which took place fairly infrequently, their lives were relatively peaceful.

With this lifestyle, parasympathetic activity of the autonomic nervous system (the rest-and-digest portion) dominated – a stark contrast to the sympathetic stimulation (fight-or-flight portion) with which most of us live in our fast-paced modern world.

As I type these words, I'm hooked up to a heart rate variability (HRV) device made by the HeartMath Institute in the USA, which specializes in researching links between the heart and brain. I do this often to help me relax as I write, as I have a habit of tensing as I type faster and faster, especially when I have an idea that I want to get on screen before I forget it. Although I enjoy writing and generally find it quite relaxing, the readout on my iPhone tells a different story.

While I have periods of parasympathetic dominance, where the rest-and-digest portion of my nervous system is dominant, for the most part it's the fight-or-flight stress portion that's running the show. I think I feel relaxed, but my nervous system is saying something else. I guess I feel relaxed relative to how I feel most of the rest of the time; however, it's clearly not the relaxed feeling of reading a book in the park on a sunny day or lying on the beach.

The Power of Natural

For many of us, stress is a habit – something we've become used to experiencing. However, thanks to the relatively calm existence enjoyed by our early ancestors, the human nervous system evolved to relax automatically when we find ourselves in natural settings.

Even a tiny green space in the middle of a bustling city can make us feel relaxed because our senses take in the plants, flowers, trees, running water, and the sounds of birds and insects. This isn't only due to the contrast between the natural setting and the busy artificial environments in which we live and work: nature has a measurable beneficial physiological effect.

Studies show that we respond rapidly to natural environments, faster even than past negative associations and memories can override them. The speed of this physiological response indicates that the preference for a natural environment is innate. Even just looking at an image of a natural setting on TV, a computer screen, or in a magazine produces a calming effect on our nerves.

Evolution is a very slow process and the human nervous system simply hasn't yet caught up with the pace of change. Our modern buildings, with their rectangular shapes and glass windows, while pleasant to look at, would be alien to our African savanna-dwelling ancestors. They don't do much for our nervous system, beyond our conscious thoughts and feelings about them. To induce a calming effect, we need to position them in natural surroundings, or at least plant natural elements in and around them.

Nature's Never-ending Patterns

Modern research is now suggesting that fractals underlie our innate preference for natural over human-made. Benoit Mandelbrot, once Sterling Professor of Mathematical Sciences at Yale, coined the word fractal from the Latin word *fractus* (meaning irregular or fragmented) and wrote about the process of roughness or self-similarity in nature.[2]

He showed that many natural things – such as coastlines, trees, and plants – that appear rough are often made up of simple patterns that repeat themselves. No matter how far inside we look, we tend to find smaller versions of the whole. This is a fundamental property of nature herself. It's how she works. And it allows the human brain and nervous system to pick out 'natural' from 'human-made.'

Indeed, anything that has formed due to a natural process, according to Mandelbrot, does so in fractal patterns – and that includes shorelines, river deltas, plant leaves, tree branches, blood vessel branches, and crystals (whether ice, salt, or quartz).

Human-made things – whether they're buildings, vehicles, or ornaments – aren't fractal. For the most part, we make straight lines and build blocky rectangles and other similar shapes in which to live and work because it costs less and it's technologically easier to achieve.

Such is our adaptation to natural environments, though, that some researchers are now suggesting that many of our mental health problems stem from the fact that most of our personal worlds are artificial. Our bodies have evolved to feel at ease with natural, organic shapes and sounds, but we live and work in artificially lit spaces with hard lines, strange smells, alien materials, and the ringing, humming, clanking, and drone of phones, air-conditioning units, and traffic.

> *We're wired to prefer trees, plants, running water, rocks, and wood over synthetic materials. As far as the human nervous system is concerned, organic beats plastic.*

Most people don't get to experience the calming effect of nature often enough. It's not necessarily the case that the human-made environments we inhabit cause our problems, but they certainly don't help. In more natural surroundings, our evolved responses would very often help us deal with issues *before* they became issues.

Natural is Restorative

Over and above the effect of a therapy itself, one of the hidden powers of complementary medicine is that treatments tend to take place in a restorative setting – one that promotes rest and rejuvenation.

A restorative therapeutic setting helps take the body from a stressed, overwhelmed, or over-stimulated state to a natural rested state. There's a natural feel to a restorative setting and it can be outdoors or indoors. Natural healing modalities also *feel* natural to us, and therein lies more of their power. People can have restorative personalities, too. Many complementary therapy practitioners have a warm, friendly, and supportive demeanor. In a session, there's no sense of urgency; the place of therapy (a person's home in many cases) typically has a nice décor and is welcoming. Often, soft music or the sounds of nature play through a speaker or can be heard outside.

Such a setting is healing in itself, before any words are spoken or any treatment given. It stimulates parasympathetic activity of the autonomic nervous system, easing stress in the body, boosting immune system activity and cardiovascular function, encouraging homeostasis, and helping the body to heal by itself.

Several years ago, while I was in the midst of a prolonged period of work-related stress, my friend Stephen Mulhearn invited me for a day of rest at Lendrick Lodge, his holistic retreat center in the Trossachs National Park, home to some of Scotland's most stunning scenery.

Stephen is a shamanic teacher and filmmaker who has led shamanic practices at Lendrick Lodge, as well as in Peru and Nepal, for more than 20 years. When I arrived, he took my phone, wallet, and car keys and immediately sent me out on an 8-mile (13-kilometer) circular walk that would take in the peak of Ben A'an, a rugged local hill, or 'mini mountain,' as it's often called.

I set out in my stressed state, and at least an hour passed before my mind began to calm and I stopped thinking about all the things I needed to do and the conflicts that existed in my workplace at the time. As I labored along the road, I was so caught up in my thoughts that I barely noticed the stunning views of Loch Venachar to my left.

Around halfway up Ben A'an, I emerged from what looked like an enchanted forest and for the first time, I started to get out of my headspace and into properly noticing my surroundings. I'd walked for two hours by then, and my mind had been on a loop, going over and over the same conversations about a couple of issues in the office. But now I began to see what was around me, and it was breathtaking!

I could see Ben Lomond, the tallest mountain in the region, and miles upon miles of lush green forest. The sun was shining and as I approached the summit of Ben A'an I experienced feelings of peace and exhilaration that I'd forgotten existed.

Would I have achieved this sense of calm while walking around a city for the same length of time? It's unlikely. I rested peacefully at the summit for a while, breathing in the panoramic views of forests, lochs, and mountains, and then slowly made my way back to Lendrick Lodge. It was the first time in a long while that I'd felt truly still and rested. All my thoughts and worries about work had disappeared. In the space of a single day, I'd been restored.

The human nervous system recognizes nature and becomes calm all by itself. It's how we're wired. The association between nature and parasympathetic activity has been ingrained over eons. No matter how hard we try to keep thinking, if we give it long enough, nature will win in the end – it will eventually overpower our busy mind and ease us into a state of peace.

A Window on Nature

Does the setting and context in which a medicine or therapy is given play a role in a patient's healing? The science shows that it can either help or hinder it. There's more to medicine than medicine.

Over the course of a year in a residential rehabilitation center in Røros, Norway, 278 coronary and pulmonary patients recovered in rooms that offered either a panoramic view of the surrounding valley and mountains or a view that was blocked by buildings.[3] Those patients with the views of nature made a faster recovery in both their mental and physical health. A blocked view of the valley and mountains, on the other hand, actually slowed the patients' rate of improvement in mental and physical health. There were also slight differences between men and women – men gained more in their mental health, and women in their physical health.

In a review of similar research, Bjørn Grinde of the Norwegian Institute of Public Health and Grete Grindal Patil of the Norwegian

University of Life Sciences concluded that an environment devoid of nature may act as a 'discord' (mismatch) with a potentially undesirable effect on health or quality of life. Being deprived of nature can be harmful.[4]

Records from a Pennsylvania hospital from 1972 to 1981 tell a similar story. Patients who had gone through cholecystectomy (removal of the gallbladder) had been assigned to rooms with windows that faced either a park or a brick wall. The patients who could see the park had shorter postoperative hospital stays, took fewer analgesics, and also had fewer negative comments in the nurses' notes.[5]

And even without a scenic view, it appears that bringing natural elements into an indoor environment can confer mental and physical health benefits.

Bringing the Outside In

Ancient Egyptian tomb paintings and surveys of the ruins of Pompeii in Italy suggest that in many cultures, plants have long been incorporated within living spaces. Today, a hypothesis called biophilia posits that humans have an innate tendency to seek connections with nature and living things.[6] In recent years, many scientific studies have looked into the effects of adding elements of nature to otherwise sterile environments.

In a study conducted by researchers at Kansas State University in the USA, 90 patients who were recovering from an appendectomy were randomized into hospital rooms with and without plants.[7] Those who recovered in the rooms containing plants needed fewer analgesics for pain – they also had lower blood pressure and heart rate and less anxiety and fatigue than those patients who recovered in rooms without plants.

And in a simulated hospital room setting in which volunteers had their pain tolerance measured, some had the test done in a normal patient room and others took it in an identical room that contained a few plants. Remarkably, this small addition of plants to the room gave the volunteers a higher tolerance for pain. They also had less activation in the fight-or-flight (stress) portion of their ANS in response to the pain.[8]

The researchers also noted that the volunteers' pain tolerance and calming of the nervous system was even greater when the room contained flowering as well as foliage plants. It wasn't just a psychological tolerance – in that they felt a bit better – rather, the brain actually responded differently to pain depending on whether or not the volunteers could see the plants.

Given that the majority of hospital patients suffer pain for some duration, it appears that the simple introduction of plants to their room would reduce that pain in many instances, depending on its severity and their condition. This intervention wouldn't make painkillers unnecessary, but patients might need fewer of them.

> *As airy-fairy as it sounds, we might find that on occasion, we could swap a couple of ibuprofen for a peace lily or a rubber plant.*

In another study, participants had their ANS response monitored while they were shown images of natural settings, such as parks, trees, rivers, or mountains, or non-natural settings, such as built-up areas. Those who saw the natural images experienced large drops in their ANS response.[9]

The Rise of Ecotherapy

Several studies have shown that doing physical exercise outdoors is more beneficial to our mental well-being than doing similar exercise indoors.[10] Of course, it's difficult to have a gym outdoors, especially if you live in a part of the world that's not always warm and sunny, but in general, when we compare running or walking outdoors in a natural setting with the same type and level of exercise indoors, outdoor exercise tends to produce bigger drops in depression, anger, and mental and emotional tension; they also make us feel more energized and revitalized.

This kind of research has given a boost to what's known as ecotherapy, which is defined as 'an intervention that improves mental and physical health and well-being by supporting people to be active outdoors.'[11] Many ecotherapists believe that a person's relationship with nature is as important as their relationships with people.

In a five-year UK project called Ecominds that was commissioned by the charity MIND and involved the NHS, universities, charities, and community groups, outdoor exercise (which not only included things like exercise in green spaces, but also growing plants) was shown to have a very healthy effect on mental health.[12] Of the participants, 62 percent reported improvements in well-being, 76 percent reported improvements in mood, and 62 percent saw improvements in their self-esteem.

A 2019 Cornell University review pointed out that there are now more than 100 quality scientific studies that demonstrate the beneficial effects of nature and green spaces on human health and well-being.[13]

With knowledge of these kinds of studies becoming more widespread, things are beginning to change. For example, in looking for ways to improve the health of NHS staff, patients, and even local communities, the NHS Forest project in the UK aims to increase access to green spaces on NHS-owned land.

The Healing Sounds of Nature

Over three sunny days in May 2017, 83 men and women took it in turns to walk around the historic Czech Republic city of Hradec Králové while wearing headphones. Scientists at the local university wanted to know if what they listened to would make them walk faster or slower. The participants all walked the same 1.1-mile (1.8-kilometer) route while being timed on stopwatches.[14]

Around a third of the participants were in a control group, so they wore headphones that didn't play any sounds – they just walked the route so the scientists could establish a baseline for how long it would take to complete.

Another third of the participants listened to birdsong while they walked, which consisted of the tweets and chirps of forest-dwelling birds, along with the sounds produced by a calm river. And the other third listened to traffic noise on their headphones – a track that had been recorded at the side of a busy road in Calcutta, India, complete with engine noises, frequent and intense loud horns, and human voices.

Listening to the forest birdsong slowed the walking pace of the volunteers in that group to an average speed of 3.4mph (5.5kph); they took longer to complete the route than the other two groups. Those listening to the noisy traffic sounds, on the other hand, walked about 8 percent faster throughout the whole route, at an average of almost 3.7mph (6kph), completing it much quicker. The walking speed of the control group was in between the two. The researchers noted that the sound of birdsong made the volunteers both mentally and physically calmer.

The route took the walkers through different sections of the city. One section contained grass, trees, buildings, and traffic, typical of a city, while other sections were similar but without buildings; a short section featured a dense oak valley without traffic. All three groups walked at their fastest pace when they were near buildings and there was traffic around, but everyone slowed their pace considerably as they walked past the dense region of oak trees. It wasn't only the sound of nature that slowed them, but also the sight of it.

Sound Effects

Other studies have also shown that the sounds of nature are hugely therapeutic. In hospitals, mechanical ventilation is an extremely common and life-saving treatment, but it can be highly distressing for the recipient and cause severe anxiety. In a university teaching hospital in the Iranian capital, Tehran, 60 patients receiving mechanical ventilation in an ICU were randomized to receive either standard care, or standard care with the addition of listening to nature-based sounds through headphones for 90 minutes.[15]

The patients could choose between the sounds of birds, a forest, a waterfall, streams, or soothing rainfall. It was found that the nature sounds had a considerable effect. While listening to the sounds and for 30 minutes afterward, the patients' anxiety levels dropped, along with agitation levels and blood pressure.

Eons of living in grasslands amid birdsong, running water, the sound of crickets, the call of wildlife, and trees swaying in the breeze conditioned the human nervous system to relax when we hear nature's voice.

> *Our nervous system is, in effect, tuned to the sounds of nature. When we hear her call, tension and stress reduce and calm takes their place.*

A double-blind randomized controlled trial of 57 mothers undergoing cesarean section conducted at Jahrom University of Medical Sciences in Iran examined the effects of nature-based sounds on the severity of their pain.[16] They were randomly assigned to three groups. The first group listened to nature-based sounds through headphones, the second group had headphones with no sound, and the third group received neither sounds nor headphones. Pain levels were significantly lower in the group who listened to the nature-based sounds.

In other research, psychologists at Stockholm University in Sweden studied the effect of different kinds of sounds on the stress responses of volunteers.[17] Participants performed a stressful mental arithmetic exercise and the researchers then measured the length of time it took for their nervous system to return to normal levels while they listened to one of four kinds of sounds: (a) natural sounds of birds singing and water in a fountain at a low volume of 50 decibels; (b) traffic noise at 80 decibels; (c) low traffic sounds at 50 decibels; or (d) the ambient noise of a ventilation system at 40 decibels (to simulate a typical office environment).

The participants' nervous systems returned to baseline levels much quicker while they listened to the nature sounds than with any of the other three kinds of sounds.

It's important to reiterate here that the sounds of nature don't just 'sound a bit relaxing,' as some skeptics assume. Rather, the sounds themselves produce direct physiological effects because of our evolutionary adaptations to them. Humans have become like tuning forks that vibrate sweetly to the sounds of nature.

Recent research indicates that different kinds of sounds affect us in different ways; however, because these studies are known only to the academics who study the subject, unsurprisingly, there's limited consensus on what kind of sounds might be of the greatest benefit.

Natural Sounds Versus Relaxing Music

Relaxing music created by musical instruments is processed differently in the brain than natural sounds. A US study by psychologists at Brandeis University in Waltham, Massachusetts, together with psychologists from the universities of Zurich, Switzerland, and Marburg, Germany, which involved 60 female volunteers, compared listening to different sounds before a stressful event.[18]

The researchers wanted to measure how quickly the participants' nervous systems would return to baseline levels depending on the type of acoustic stimulation. One group listened to relaxing music, and the second group to the sound of swirling water; to serve as a control, a third group didn't listen to any sounds.

Measurements were taken of salivary amylase, an enzyme in the saliva that's increased by ANS activity during stress. These levels returned to baseline fastest in the group who listened to relaxing music – faster even than in the group who listened to nature sounds (swirling water). However, the nature sounds group had lower cortisol levels and their heart rate variability, a measure of ANS activity, returned to normal faster than in the other two groups.

The study suggested that both relaxing music and nature sounds relax us, but they do so via *different* biological pathways. The human nervous system has adapted to natural sounds over eons, so we'd expect these to impact more ancient systems in the brain and body, such as those that produce stress hormones and regulate heart rate. But relaxing music is a more recent introduction to our nervous system so we might expect it to impact the brain and body in slightly different, albeit still relaxing, ways, because relaxing music is designed to be, well, relaxing.

Relaxing music, which is typically played in many complementary therapy settings, can be immensely beneficial in a conventional medicine setting too. Severely ill patients experience a great deal of fear and anxiety in hospital – due to their diagnosis, the procedure they have to undergo, fear of progress in recovery, fear of disability, fear of death, or helplessness and loss of control.

A review of 26 randomized controlled trials on the use of relaxing music with coronary heart disease patients showed that the music produced overall reductions in anxiety, heart rate, respiratory rate, blood pressure, and quality of sleep following their surgery.[19]

Empathy Can Heal

'I don't have time for empathy,' a GP once told me. It wasn't meant unkindly; in fact, he said it with a hint of sadness. His practice was so busy that he was almost always behind schedule and he found this stressful. Showing empathy to his patients, something that came naturally to him, only put him further behind as it led them to open up more.

Over time, he'd learned to shut himself off a little, to become more direct and clinical. But it was taking a toll on his mental health. He longed for a different kind of medical practice, one in which he could sit with a patient and listen to what *really* ailed them. Much of the time, he told me, patients just needed to talk. 'If I let them do that,' he remarked, 'I wouldn't need to prescribe as many drugs.'

Complementary therapies tend to allow longer interactions between practitioner and patient than in a conventional medicine setting, so there's more time for empathy, and more time for a patient to benefit from it. For a large number of people, for a lot of what ails them, empathy is a tonic they need more than a physical medicine.

> *Sometimes, when the spirit is soothed with a little extra care, the body returns to balance all by itself.*

A smile, kind eyes, a listening ear while they communicate their pains – physical, emotional, and spiritual – stimulates a patient's natural healing processes.

Recent research backs up that GP's sentiments. A doctor who shows empathy heals more patients than one who is more forthright and clinical. Studies show that patients of high-empathy doctors are more likely to take on board what they're advised to do and are more likely to complete their full course of treatment.

High-Empathy Doctors

In a review of the published literature on the role of empathy on patient satisfaction, adherence to treatment, and patient outcomes, researchers at Radboud University Nijmegen Medical Center in the Netherlands stated that 'empathy in the patient-physician communication in general practice is of unquestionable importance.'[20] They reported that empathy lowers anxiety and distress levels in patients and that it delivers significantly better clinical outcomes.

A number of studies now show that doctor empathy even has a significant impact on a patient's immune system. In one study, more than 700 patients treated for symptoms of the common cold received either a regular consultation or an empathy-enhanced consultation.[21] Empathy substantially lifted the patients' immune responses, and their recovery times were almost 50 percent faster than in those who received a lower-empathy consultation.

Similarly, a study of 175 prostate cancer patients found that those treated by a high-empathy doctor had higher levels of NK (natural killer) cells and that these increased significantly over a three-month period compared with patients treated with doctors who showed less empathy.[22]

In fact, empathy benefits patients suffering from a range of conditions. In studies, people with diabetes have been shown to have far fewer acute metabolic complications, including diabetic ketoacidosis,[23] while cancer patients had a higher quality of life; for them, empathy was also protective against depression.[24] Patients with asthma,[25] Crohn's disease,[26] and ulcerative colitis[27] all had lower anxiety levels, better sleep quality, and lower inflammation levels when shown empathy by their doctors.

Empathy can make a person feel calm, but it can also stimulate the production of oxytocin – which has been shown to impact cardiovascular function by reducing blood pressure via the stimulation of nitric oxide release – boost immune function, and affect the rate of healing of wounds, even after surgery. For these additional reasons, empathy alone, before any prescription or treatment is given, can heal.

The Active Ingredients

For any type of therapy, whether drug or alternative, scientific studies tend to try to isolate what *works*. This is called the active ingredient, and to identify it, scientists remove any other factor that might be contributing to the outcome. The idea is to discover precisely what it is about the therapy or drug – the *single thing* that's doing the business – and it's all about the active ingredient; everything else is irrelevant.

It wasn't always that way. The first hospitals in Europe were set in monastic communities in which a garden was considered essential and was believed to support the healing process. In modern medicine, we've largely forgotten that nature is our ally. A century or so ago, almost all medicines were plant extracts; some are still in use today, such as aspirin from willow bark, quinine from cinchona bark, and morphine from the opium poppy. But drug discovery has moved in a new direction.

The process of pharmaceutical drug development typically begins when a chemical substance is isolated from a plant that's known to confer some medicinal benefits. The substance is identified after testing the hundreds of ingredients in a leaf, section of bark, or piece of root. Then, different versions of it are made by making tiny alterations to the chemical structure until an 'analogue' is found that's more potent than the original natural substance for the intended purpose.

To picture how this works, imagine a piece of Plasticine molded into the shape of a tree with several branches. Now, snip off half of a branch from the top right of the tree and stick it at an angle halfway along a branch near the bottom left. In drug discovery, this new shape (chemical structure) would be one analogue of the original.

Several hundred (or thousand) analogues are usually made by swapping and snipping different branches and adding new ones, and all are tested until one is found that's more potent than the natural substance isolated from the plant. It's a logical process that's produced some powerful and life-saving medicines.

The analogue eventually becomes the drug that's prescribed to patients for a medical condition. It's the active ingredient – the thing that does the curing or the relieving of symptoms. Other substances, known as excipients, are added to make a tablet, such as those that improve its absorption or how well it dissolves, but these are considered inert. The only ingredient that has any actual clinical effect – the active ingredient – is the drug.

Non-Drug Active Ingredients

Drugs, however, aren't used in complementary medicine, and since the only notion of an active ingredient we've had for the last century or so has been chemical, anything else sounds woo-woo. But complementary treatments have active ingredients too, only not in the chemical sense, unless they're herbal, Chinese, or Ayurvedic medicines.

One of these active ingredients is the treatment itself; then there's the setting and the sounds in which it's given, and the empathy of the therapist and how they communicate with the patient – the words they use and, importantly, *how* they speak them. There are other ingredients, too, and together, they all contribute to the restoration of wellness in a patient.

These active ingredients exist in a GP surgery or a hospital ward too, but for the past century our focus has been largely on the active ingredient of a drug, and we've completely missed (or some would say, forgotten) the simple value of a kind, reassuring smile, a compassionate personality, a warm and welcoming room, and a window view of nature through which the songs of birds echo.

Sometimes, especially with potent drugs for acute and other very serious conditions, one active ingredient dominates and is clearly the most important; however, we've come to believe that this is the case in *every* scenario, which makes us suspicious of anything that isn't a pill, an injection, or surgery. But it's not.

As we saw in Chapter 1, where patient recovery was compared against the way the doctor communicated, an empathetic, reassuring, or enthusiastic doctor will heal patients faster than a more clinical or uncertain doctor, even when they prescribe exactly the same drugs.

Similarly, a warmly decorated room will help patients with their mental and physical health better than a plain one. And a room that contains plants, especially flowering ones, will speed up recovery, calm the nervous system, and reduce pain. These are all active ingredients. Patients will also sometimes respond better when the doctor is wearing glasses, simply because they associate glasses with intelligence.

The Built-in Placebo Effect

There's a contribution, large or small, from a drug or therapy, but there's a contribution from the environment in which it takes place, too, as well as from the way the therapist communicates. There are multiple active ingredients in every scenario, some lending more weight at times and some lending less, but all of them contributing to a restoration of wellness.

> **All active ingredients contribute to the totality of any treatment or therapy, whether conventional or complementary.**

In many instances, the setting, the sounds, the pleasantness of the practitioner, and the amount of time they've set aside to work with you, which is usually around an hour in a complementary setting compared with 10 minutes in a doctor's consulting room, is just what you need. Sometimes, a little empathy and a good rest will do a patient a world of good. We need to expand our view of what medicine is. This is the 21st century – medicine is more than a tablet, injection, or surgery.

Skeptics dismiss the active ingredients I've outlined as *just* placebo, but we need to expand our concepts. In an interview with *Time* magazine, Ted Kaptchuk, Harvard Professor of Medicine and one of the world's leading authorities on the placebo effect, said that 'a therapy's built-in placebo effect can be considered a distinct aspect of its efficacy, and that placebo-induced benefits should be promoted, not dismissed.'[28]

This built-in placebo effect can be the setting, the sounds, empathy, and so on, and we should encourage it, not try to delete it from the equation. When we ignore the setting and context it reduces the potency of any treatment; in a sense, we use the environment and context against ourselves.

A Lifestyle Prescription

It's estimated that more than 70 percent of all doctor visits are stress related. Given this, each year millions of people could benefit from restorative environments and complementary treatments in these environments, offering a potentially huge saving to our overstretched healthcare services. Time and cost could be focused more on people who are seriously ill, who do require more expensive or complex medications and surgical interventions, and who might not otherwise be able to receive the treatment they need because so much is spent on people who simply need a good rest.

Things *are* changing, though. In the USA, Integrative Medicine, which integrates conventional Western medicine with varying complementary practices, is becoming increasingly recognized as valid and effective. In fact, the US Congress has spent billions in establishing the National Center for Complementary and Integrative Health (NCCIH) to research its usefulness and safety.

The NCCIH classifies therapies into five groups: (1) biologically based, which includes herbs, supplements, and diet;

(2) manipulative and body-based systems, such as massage, chiropractic, and osteopathy; (3) mind–body medicine, including meditation, yoga, and tai chi; (4) alternative medical systems, including Chinese medicine, Ayurvedic medicine, and homeopathy; and (5) energy therapies, including reiki, therapeutic touch, and others. This has been driven by interest from both the public and health professionals and health institutions who are recognizing the effectiveness of many of these treatments.

Things are evolving in the UK, too. A 2018 survey found that 16 percent of the English adult population, around 9 million people, have now visited a complementary practitioner for reiki, massage, osteopathy, chiropractic, acupuncture, or one of many other healing modalities.[29]

A growing number of UK medical doctors now embrace 'lifestyle' or 'progressive' medicine, appreciating that patients benefit from a good diet and exercise as well as from the medicine they're prescribed. If a condition isn't serious, some of these doctors even prefer to treat a patient's lifestyle first, offering interventions for dietary, lifestyle, and even stress management that might reduce the need for drugs.

Dr. Rangan Chatterjee, GP, author, and host of the highly influential podcast series 'Feel Better, Live More' writes, 'I focus on finding the root cause of diseases and help my patients make their illnesses disappear. This means that as a doctor I focus on all of you, not just the symptoms. I don't treat the disease. I treat the person. The majority of patients don't need a pill, they need a lifestyle prescription.'[30]

Dr. Punam Krishan is a GP at a practice on the outskirts of Glasgow in Scotland, a trustee and regional director for the

British Society of Lifestyle Medicine, and presenter of the BBC series *Laid Bare*, about lifestyle medicine. Like Dr. Chatterjee, and a growing number of doctors who take lifestyle very seriously, she views five lifestyle-based active ingredients in doctor treatments as important beyond any drug prescribed. These five components that influence health are physical activity, nutrition, community, sleep, and stress.

Dr. Krishan estimates that during her nine years as a GP, 70–80 percent of chronic diseases presenting to primary care, including heart disease, type 2 diabetes, stroke, and even some cancers, were related to lifestyle habits, and these are reversible. So important are these active ingredients that she regularly takes patients on a tour of the local supermarket and teaches them which foods are healthy, which ones should be avoided, and even how to read food labels.[31]

CHAPTER 5

Reiki

The word *heal* has its roots in various cultures: it's derived from *hælan* in Old English (or Anglo-Saxon), meaning 'to restore to sound health'; from *hailjan* in Proto-Germanic, meaning 'to make whole,' and from the Scots *hale*, meaning 'to heal.' More generally, it means 'to make healthy, whole, or sound; to restore to health.'

As we discussed in previous chapters, anything that helps to make a person whole or helps restore them to health, then, is healing. This can mean the sights and sounds of nature, relaxing music, the warm smile of an empathetic doctor, or the gentle manner of a complementary therapist. It can also mean good nutrition, exercise, meditation, sleep, rest, and releasing repressed negative emotions. It can mean herbal supplements, vitamins, and it can be prescribed drugs or surgery.

Over the past century, we've come to believe almost entirely that healing can only result from drugs or surgery, and as a consequence, most other approaches to healing are written off as pseudoscience. However, there's a growing amount of evidence for the effectiveness of all the aforementioned routes to wholeness and sound health.

The Rise of Complementary Medicine

In the USA, the top 15 academic hospitals, including Duke, Yale, and Johns Hopkins, now offer reiki, Therapeutic Touch (TT), Chinese herbal therapy, massage, homeopathy, hypnotherapy, meditation, yoga, aromatherapy, art therapy, acupuncture, biofeedback, guided imagery, and many other complementary therapies.[1]

Many leading hospitals in the UK, Europe, the USA, and around the world now have integrative medicine centers for the purpose of treating the patient in a more holistic way, offering them lifestyle advice, complementary therapies, and a restorative setting.

In the USA, the Institute of Lifestyle Medicine, founded at Spaulding Rehabilitation Hospital and Harvard Medical School, has a goal to transform the practice of clinical care through lifestyle medicine. It conducts research and offers education to physicians and other healthcare practitioners that guides the treatments offered to patients in a holistic way.

The British Society of Lifestyle Medicine in the UK has a similar goal. Its members are doctors based throughout the country who recognize that there's more to medicine than prescribing pills, and that many interventions can be avoided altogether with various preventative lifestyle habits. The Royal London Hospital for Integrated Medicine in London, part of the University College London Hospitals and NHS Foundation Trust, states that they 'consider the whole person and their environment in the quest for optimal health and well-being.'[2]

Some hospitals have now constructed spa-like facilities to help create a holistic and restorative environment that's conducive to the use of these complementary therapies. Despite attracting a small amount of criticism, these settings alone facilitate healing over and above any practices that take place within them.

A survey conducted by the American Hospital Association asked such hospitals why they've created these facilities and offer complementary therapies and found that 85 percent said that it was due to patient demand. And patient demand isn't the only factor. The scientific evidence speaks for itself.[3]

A large study tracked more than 6,500 cardiovascular patients admitted to a large US hospital over a three-year period who had received some form of integrative medicine; this included mind–body energy therapies, bodywork, traditional Chinese medicine, and combination therapies.[4] After receiving one or more of the treatments, patients averaged a 47 percent reduction in pain and a 55 percent reduction in anxiety. An analysis of more than 1,800 oncology patients at the same hospital who also received some form of integrative medicine found that they had enjoyed similar reductions in pain and anxiety.[5]

Reiki's Healing Touch

Reiki is one of the 'energy healing' techniques offered at many large hospitals. It's a relaxing form of therapy that's applied through gentle, noninvasive touch, with the practitioner laying their hands either on or just above specific regions of the body. In this chapter, we'll look at the results of several scientific studies on reiki, as well as some of the reasons why the technique can be effective.

There are other forms of energy healing, among them Therapeutic Touch, pranic healing, qigong, craniosacral therapy, chakra balancing and Johrei, but I've focused on reiki for two main reasons. First, because it's one of the most criticized complementary therapies and is frequently dismissed as quackery, and second, because it's also one of the most scientifically tested.

The word reiki is composed of two Japanese words: *rei*, meaning 'hidden force or higher power' and *ki*, meaning 'life energy.' Reiki is believed to have been developed in Japan in the early 20th century by a Zen Buddhist named Mikau Usui as he undertook a 21-day fast and penance on Mount Kurama. The story goes that he became enlightened with the knowledge of reiki on the 21st day and was healed. On his return to his village, he set up a clinic and began offering reiki freely to people.

Conventional medicine is complex and requires a thorough understanding of the workings of the human body and an in-depth knowledge of different disease processes and available treatments. Reiki, however, doesn't require this type of knowledge. The goal of reiki is to assist the body's own restorative processes, so the treatment has spiritual and emotional undertones.

> *Reiki is holistic and makes more use of the*
> *active ingredients of setting, context, and*
> *empathy than does conventional medicine.*

Reiki typically activates the parasympathetic nervous system,[6] which then aids the immune system by relieving some of the stress pressure on it. This alone helps to shift many people in the direction of healing.

The Evidence for Reiki

Reiki is fast becoming accepted in UK hospitals and as a private practice. Alongside this are a growing number of scientific studies that show it can be very effective. Several have demonstrated that reiki reduces pain, anxiety, depression, and even blood pressure in patients suffering from a range of medical conditions or who have experienced various interventions – including cancer, knee replacement, hysterectomy, hemodialysis, back pain, and many others.

For example, a 2018 meta-analysis of four randomized controlled studies into the use of reiki for reducing pain over a range of conditions concluded that it produced statistically significant reductions in pain.[7] And a 2019 *British Medical Journal Supportive & Palliative Care* review concluded that 'reiki therapy is useful for relieving pain, decreasing anxiety/depression, and improving quality of life in several conditions.'[8]

In many research studies, reiki is compared with mimic (also called sham) reiki, in which an actor mimics the movements and hand positions of a trained reiki practitioner. The idea is to model a drug-placebo comparison, with mimic reiki considered to be the placebo; however, if mimic reiki is done in the same restorative setting as real reiki it will almost always stimulate parasympathetic activity and produce results, so the comparison isn't entirely appropriate. Even so, reiki typically shows better results than mimic reiki.

In a study led by researchers at Celal Bayar University School of Health Services in Turkey, for example, 45 women who had had a cesarean section were given either reiki or mimic reiki over the incision area for 15 minutes following the surgery.[9] Some women didn't receive either reiki or mimic reiki, so that a full comparison could be made.

Two treatments were given, within 24 and 48 hours of the surgery and within 4–8 hours following administration of standard analgesics. Reiki produced a sizable reduction in pain, systolic blood pressure, and even average breathing rate compared with mimic reiki and the comparison group. The women who received reiki also needed fewer painkillers and could endure pain for longer before requesting them.

Reiki for Cancer Patients

A growing number of cancer patients now seek some form of complementary medicine, including reiki. Some try it to manage their pain, others to help manage stress, anxiety, or depression, and others still use it to manage the side effects of their treatments. A 2017 pilot study at the radiotherapy department of the National Cancer Institute in Rome, Italy, studied the latter.[10] It examined the effects of reiki on patients with head-neck neoplasia who were undergoing radiotherapy; it was found to be highly effective at reducing the side effects of the treatment.

Fatigue is a very common side effect in patients receiving cancer treatments. A small study involving 16 cancer patients compared daily reiki treatments with patients who rested during those times. Significantly, fatigue was reduced in the patients who received reiki, but not in those who rested. Those who received reiki also enjoyed significant improvements in their quality of life; they also reported reductions in pain and anxiety levels compared with those in the resting group.[11]

A seven-day phase II trial looked at quality of life and painkilling analgesic use in 24 advanced cancer patients.[12] Reiki was given for 90 minutes around one hour after the patients' afternoon analgesic dose on days one and four; the patients who received reiki were compared with those who didn't. The patients who had reiki had much improved pain control following each treatment. There was no change in analgesic use, but given that the reiki was offered after the analgesic, this might be expected.

Children respond well to reiki too. A small study of nine children with cancer who were receiving stem cell treatment as their main intervention also received 88 reiki sessions between them (around 10 sessions each).[13] The object of the study was to see if reiki could reduce their pain. And it did – significantly so. The study authors even recommended that reiki could be formally introduced to help reduce pain in children with cancer.

In a 396-bed academic tertiary medical center in the US state of New Hampshire, private patients were told they could request reiki or massage, or they were sometimes referred to the healing arts team and received either reiki or a massage.[14] Some of these patients were cancer sufferers and others had various other conditions.

Over a period of five years, scientists assessed the health outcomes of a large number of patients attending the center who received either a single reiki session or a single massage session. They charted levels of pain, nausea, fatigue, anxiety, depression, and overall well-being, depending on which symptoms each person had.

Even with just the single reiki session, patients experienced immediate relief in symptoms of pain, nausea, fatigue, anxiety, and depression as well as increases in overall well-being. The levels of relief were similar for reiki and massage in both cancer patients and non-cancer patients, and reiki was a little more effective than massage in improving fatigue and anxiety.

These patients could have received similar relief from drugs, of course, but the point is that drugs weren't necessary. Reiki or massage, combined with the restorative setting, were enough of a tonic for them.

Reiki Following Surgery

A study compared pain and anxiety levels in women after they underwent abdominal hysterectomies.[15] Ten women received standard nursing care plus three 30-minute reiki sessions over three days and they were compared with 12 women who received standard nursing care alone, without the reiki. The women who had the reiki had much less pain and anxiety and they also requested fewer analgesics than the women who didn't receive the reiki.

Researchers at the US universities of Arizona and Drexel, and at the Center for Reiki Research in Michigan, conducted a blinded controlled pilot study of 46 patients undergoing a knee replacement at Abington Memorial Hospital in Pennsylvania.[16] They measured the effect of reiki on pain, anxiety, and blood pressure and found that all levels dropped following reiki treatments. Patients had either received reiki or mimic reiki treatment, but those who received the reiki had the biggest reductions in pain, anxiety, and blood pressure.

A similar study took place at Bryn Mawr Hospital in Pennsylvania with patients undergoing surgery for total knee replacement.[17]

Twenty-three patients received reiki treatments and 20 were in a comparison group. Pain was assessed before and after each reiki treatment in the preoperative area, the post-anesthesia care unit, and on each of three postoperative days. All the reiki sessions resulted in significant reductions in pain levels before and following surgery, although not in the post-anesthesia care unit.

The results of the study were so significant, and feedback from the patients had been so positive, that the hospital soon established a dedicated reiki program for which 10 nurses were trained and certified in reiki.

Pain is a significant problem for patients undergoing hemodialysis, where a dialysis machine is used to clean the blood. In a 2018 study, 15 patients were given reiki for 20 minutes twice a week for four weeks, and then had their levels of pain, fatigue, and depression assessed; these were all found to be significantly reduced as a result of the reiki sessions.[18]

As is sometimes the case due to the negative perception of complementary treatments, the medical staff were initially quite reluctant to allow the reiki, but they quickly observed that it didn't interfere with their workflow in any way. By the end of the study, having witnessed the beneficial results and responses in the patients, the staff agreed that reiki could easily be integrated into their practice settings.

Other Reiki Studies

Some studies compare reiki with other practices that are in established use for certain chronic conditions. Often, they show that reiki can be just as effective as these treatments, and even better than prescribed drugs in many situations. For example, a study led by researchers at Zabol University of Medical Sciences in Iran compared reiki against physiotherapy and drug treatment for relieving lower back pain and improving the activities of daily living in patients with an intervertebral disc hernia.[19]

Sixty patients were randomly assigned to receive reiki, physiotherapy, or drug treatment. Both reiki and physiotherapy significantly reduced levels of pain and were much more effective than drug treatment. The overall painkilling effect was quite similar between the reiki and physiotherapy groups and those patients also improved in their ability to carry out normal daily activities as a consequence.

And in a room at New England University within the College of Nursing and Health Professions, community-dwelling older adults who were experiencing pain, depression, and anxiety were given a 45-minute reiki treatment each Friday for eight consecutive weeks.[20] The room had soft lighting and relaxing music was played. After that period, the subjects' pain levels and mental health were compared with others in the community who hadn't received reiki. For many of the individuals, reiki had worked absolute wonders, and they enjoyed significant reductions in pain, depression, and anxiety.

Reiki and Music

I've pointed out that soft lighting and relaxing music were used in this study as a reminder that complementary treatments such as reiki generally have multiple active ingredients. We can isolate the therapy from these if we wish, but that would be taking the therapy out of its natural setting.

Some critics of reiki do believe, though, that these effects are simply due to the fact that relaxing music is usually played during a session and any benefits reported are down to that music. It's an active ingredient, after all. But it would be a mistake to assume that it's the *only* one.

Skeptics insist that reiki does nothing other than relax the recipient, which partially misses the point, and that multiple active ingredients contribute to healing. Also, this belief is based merely on the common sense assumption that relaxing music relaxes us, without any knowledge of the scientific studies on the calming effect of natural sounds that we looked at in the previous chapter.

However, many reiki treatments are given without music, especially when they take place in a clinical setting, and they still produce excellent results. At Kennesaw State University in Georgia, USA, a study of people living with HIV addressed this by comparing music alone with music plus reiki. People living with HIV often look to complementary medicine practices to help relieve stress, anxiety, and pain, and also as a means to improve their overall health.[21]

This was a pilot study involving 37 participants who were randomly distributed into a music group or a music-plus-reiki group for six weeks. After the six weeks, and again four weeks further on, those in the music-plus-reiki group were in significantly less pain and feeling much less stressed than those in the group who listened to relaxing music alone. Reiki provided clear and significant benefits over and above the effect of music.

Real Reiki and Mimic Reiki

There are, of course, some studies that show reiki to be less effective. One such example, conducted at the University of Birmingham in the UK, was a 12-week study involving 207 adults with type 2 diabetes, in which 93 received reiki, 88 received mimic reiki (the placebo form of reiki discussed earlier), and 26 received the usual care without the reiki or mimic reiki.[22]

Reiki treatments were of 25 minutes duration and given twice in the first week and then once a week for the following 11 weeks. Pain levels reduced in the reiki and mimic reiki groups but not in the usual care group. Walking distance improved in both the reiki and mimic reiki groups too, but not in the usual care group. Both reiki and mimic reiki were shown to work.

In the mimic reiki group were actors trained to accurately mimic reiki masters in their style of practice. They reproduced the pleasant attitude, demeanor, and confident movements of reiki practitioners as they made their fake reiki movements. The setting and context was the same for both the reiki and mimic reiki.

It's not surprising that the mimic reiki delivered significant benefits, given that it provided some important active ingredients. It's easy to jump to the conclusion, as some skeptics did, that the study showed that reiki doesn't work. But once more, this overlooks the fact that multiple active ingredients contribute to a healing effect.

Indeed, although the study concluded that there was no significant difference in efficacy between reiki and mimic reiki, its authors added that given the strength of the results for both these groups, it demonstrated the important power of a 'sustained partnership' between the healthcare provider and the patient. In other words, they acknowledged that empathy and caring interaction were active ingredients in the reduction in pain.

Why Session Length Matters

As demonstrated by the earlier example of mimic reiki, the study from Celal Bayar University, most other studies *do* show a difference between real and mimic reiki. So, what was different in this particular study? Well, in the majority of the studies where reiki is found to be effective, treatments were 60 or 90 minutes in duration, not 25 minutes, as was the case here. The study would have offered a better test if the reiki sessions had been of this length.

A typical reiki session length gives plenty of time for a person to relax and benefit from the treatment. Plus, the hand positions that reiki practitioners are trained to use typically take longer than 25 minutes to work through. Shorter reiki sessions can of course be beneficial, but it might be that 25 minutes isn't long enough to see a difference between reiki and mimic reiki because the latter is providing benefits too.

Certainly, the meta-analyses and randomized controlled trials reported in the past few years have strongly asserted that reiki is effective at reducing pain and the symptoms of anxiety and depression.

The Science of Reiki

Contrary to popular belief, a reiki practitioner doesn't *heal* a patient in the sense that they fix something that's wrong with them. According to the US National Center for Complementary and Integrative Health, the goal of the practitioner is to direct energy to help facilitate the person's *own* healing response. In this way, a reiki healer assists the patient to heal themselves.

Reiki is classified as a biofield energy therapy, as are Therapeutic Touch (TT), Healing Touch (HT), pranic healing, qigong, Johrei, and others. While the term biofield might sound woo-woo, it's simply an electric or magnetic field – a field of energy or information – that's produced by a biological organism. Therefore, we all have a biofield, on account of the movement of ions in and out of our cells.

> *It's believed that reiki helps balance a person's energy field, or biofield, and as that occurs, it helps to facilitate their own healing responses.*

There's a simple way to visualize the way reiki and other biofield energy therapies are believed to work. A plate of hot food gives off heat. The temperature of the environment around the plate is correlated with the temperature of the food, and that's why the air close to the food feels warm. But if we altered the temperature 'field' (the area of heat) around the food, it would impact on the food itself. So we could cool the food by cooling the environment around it or we could make it warmer by placing it in a hot environment.

In biofield energy therapies, the idea is to work with the energy field that surrounds the human body in the understanding that it's correlated with the body's internal state. Changes in the biofield are therefore believed to induce changes in the organism (human body) that produces the field.

Energy on Energy

All biological organisms owe their very existence to electric or magnetic fields; for example, the heart generates an electric field that regulates its beats. But at a more fundamental level, let's consider what happens when you sit on a chair. Clearly, you feel the chair and you don't fall through it, but that's not because there's any real physical contact between your rear and the chair.

The atoms that make up your rear have a nucleus of protons and neutrons that's surrounded by a cloud of electrons in varying quantum states. The electrons generate an electric field, just as a magnet generates a magnetic field that you can feel when you place another magnet close to it. The same is true of the atoms that make up the chair. When you sit on the chair, the electrons in your rear push against the electrons on the seat.

We just think of it as 'butt on seat' because that's what it feels like; however, sitting squeezes together the electric fields of the approximately million trillion trillion atoms in the chair and they subsequently push back against the electric fields of the million trillion trillion atoms in your posterior, creating an upward force that balances with your weight. This is why you don't fall through the chair. It's energy on energy, electric field on electric field.

We feel the push of the atoms that make up the chair as something solid, but the push is electrical, not physical. The physical touch we feel is how the brain processes the force between the two interacting fields. And it's always done that, so we naturally grow to recognize the sensation as physical touch. But it's energy on energy.

We're so used to thinking of things in solid physical terms that the idea of some form of 'energy,' even if it's electric or magnetic, having an effect on the body sounds mystical. So we tend to be skeptical of it. Understanding it in the way I've just outlined can help us comprehend the basis of why reiki may work. Some of its effects may also include an active ingredient of 'energy on energy' – that is, the electric or magnetic field of a healer's heart impacting on that of a patient.

Healer Heal Thyself

As I touched on earlier, the heart beats rhythmically, but there's a natural variation between the beats that's known as heart rate variability, or HRV. Typically, the heart speeds up a little when we breathe in and slows down a little when we breathe out. This is due to the signals from the two branches of the autonomic nervous system (ANS). The in breath activates the sympathetic branch and the out breath activates the parasympathetic branch.

The average time between beats on the in breath and out breath is our HRV. For example, if there was 1 second between each beat on the in breath and 1.1 seconds between each beat on the out breath, the HRV would be 0.1 seconds (1.1 minus 1), or 100 ms (milliseconds), as it's usually reported.

The HeartMath Institute in the USA has demonstrated how HRV is influenced by different emotional states.[23] Positive states such as appreciation tend to increase it, while negative states such as stress and anxiety tend to decrease it. The increase is because positive emotional states tend to feel relaxing and this causes an increase in activity of the parasympathetic portion of the autonomic nervous system.

A smooth speeding up and slowing down of the heart as we breathe is referred to as coherence, where the two ANS branches (sympathetic and parasympathetic) smoothly switch from one being dominant to the other being dominant. A jagged, erratic change on the other hand is referred to as incoherence, where essentially the two branches of the ANS aren't so much in sync.

When the two branches are in sync, an HRV waveform, when viewed on a computer screen, moves smoothly up and down like a sine wave, while a jagged, erratic pattern indicates that both branches are trying to work at the same time – it's as if you're both stimulated and relaxed at the same time; as if you're trying to relax but your nervous system is still agitated.

I use a HeartMath Institute device in some of my meditation practices because it's a very clear way of receiving biofeedback. The pattern of the waveform on my iPhone screen and the score the software gives for each second of coherence is an indication of the steadiness of my breath and the calmness of my emotional state.

I've noticed that when I feel relaxed and calm, or positive, inspired, or uplifted, the wave is usually smooth, and its height is greatest when I feel positive or inspired. But when I feel stressed or anxious, the wave resembles the top of a jagged mountain range. When I see this pattern, it encourages me to concentrate on relaxing.

The Heart's Magnetic Field

The electric field of the heart, which an ECG measures, is about 60 times greater in amplitude (strength) than the electric field of the brain, which we measure with an EEG. The heart also has a magnetic field that's about 100 times larger than the brain's magnetic field. The heart generates the largest magnetic field, in fact, of any organ in the body. A SQUID-based magnetometer (Superconducting Quantum Interference Device) will typically detect the heart's magnetic field at a distance of about 3 feet (1 meter) from a person.

The heart's magnetic field is a consequence of the way electric current moves through and around the organ as it flows into and out of heart muscle cells. This electric current is referred to as a bioelectric current; it's generated from the ions in and around cells and its source is therefore biochemical.

How does a person's emotional state affect this bioelectric current? Through the impact of mental and emotional states on blood flow and on stress hormone levels and other substances that are involved in the movement of ions in and out of cells. Positive states like happiness, joy, compassion, or gratitude tend to extend the heart's magnetic field while negative states such as stress, anxiety, or fear tend to contract it.

How a Reiki Healer's State Affects a Client

The question that's relevant to reiki is: will the magnetic field that emanates from a reiki practitioner's heart, which in turn is affected by their state, impact the client in the way that biofield therapies are believed to work? If it does, then the emotional state of the practitioner is of the utmost importance when they give a healing session because their state will influence not only the size but also the coherence of their own heart's magnetic field.

Thus, might a reiki healer, through empathy or a calm presence, exert a calming and beneficial effect on a patient? And might a stressed or agitated healer have the opposite effect? This is quite likely.

Over and above the words we speak to each other, which is an obvious means by which one person's state impacts that of another, there are two distinct ways that a person's state can impact another's and both are relevant in any therapy situation, whether it's a reiki practitioner's room or a medical doctor's consulting room. One is through the effect of the heart's magnetic field, but the other is more direct and very relevant in all healing settings – via mirror neurons.

1) Mirror Neurons

Most of us have had the direct experience of feeling stressed around a stressed person, and it's likely that we've felt someone's calming presence. Principally, this happens due to the mirror neuron system (MNS) in the brain, which facilitates what's known as emotional contagion – the transference of emotional states between people.

Emotional contagion happens every day, in almost every interaction we have with others, mostly without us noticing. In fact, studies suggest that as much as 15–25 percent of most people's average emotional state over a period of time is due to the emotions they've 'caught' from others.[24]

Emotional Contagion

Here's how emotional contagion works. Say you're hanging out with a friend who is feeling happy. Their face exhibits their state – it communicates it non-verbally – but while this is happening, your MNS mirrors the movements of your friend's facial muscles, like a video camera following a person's movements. Each time they smile, your smile muscle brain regions become activated and this causes you to smile involuntarily.

As a result, the longer you spend with your friend, the more you'll smile when they smile – not necessarily because you agree with them, but because your MNS is stimulating your smile muscles to mirror theirs.

This activation of your smile muscles also activates the emotional centers of your brain that correspond with those muscles. This means that you also start to feel how your friend feels. If they feel genuinely happy, you'll tend to feel happier. I say genuinely, because if they're faking their emotional state, your MNS picks that up too. It's part of the intuition you feel about certain people when you're around them.

Sometimes, despite appearances, you get a feeling that someone who is smiling is actually sad; this is because your MNS picks up micro movements of their facial muscles – which occur over just a few thousandths of a second – that betray how they're really feeling. And other times, despite what a person says, you get the sense that they're not telling you the whole story.

This is one of the reasons why reiki treatments are more effective than mimic reiki treatments. Reiki practitioners enter the profession because they want to help people, so they're genuinely in a state that's conducive to the healing of their client. A mimic practitioner in a study is faking it – they're just going through the motions of the physical movements. Some of them may genuinely feel empathy for the person they're working on, of course, but on the whole, mimic reiki practitioners typically won't feel empathy to the same degree as that of an experienced practitioner whose vocation is to help others.

> *Reiki practitioners talk of being a 'channel' of reiki, in the sense that it flows through them to the patient, and it's almost certain that this occurs.*

The practitioner's awareness of the meaning of reiki symbols – for example, power (*cho ku rei*) or harmony (*sei hei ki*) – will subtly alter their expressions, most likely enough to transfer this state to the patient, given that the MNS takes emotional snapshots down to just a few thousandths of a second. In this way, the practitioner does allow reiki to flow through them to the patient.

The MNS allows us to catch the full range of emotional states from other people; however, the amount we catch at any one time is related to our general tendency for empathy, or our emotional connection with that particular person. The more we like, admire, or look up to a person, or the more empathy they show that causes us to feel open to them, the more likely we are to catch their emotions.

In any setting where a bond is formed, however temporary, emotional contagion takes place. The direction in which it flows – that is, who is the sender and who is the receiver – depends on who is the stronger expresser of their emotions.

We all know people who exude a state of calm: they wear it all over their face and body. When you're in their company, if they exude calm more than you express stress, then their calm state will win and the situation will tend toward one that's calmer. If you feel more stress than they feel calm, on the other hand, then your state will win and they'll either become a little stressed or leave the room. In this context, then, a healer isn't only a person who knows medicine. A healer is someone who can maintain a state of calm in the face of someone else's anxiety, fear, stress, or discomfort.

The Healer as an Active Ingredient

Now consider this in the context of an interaction between a doctor and a patient, or a reiki healer and a client. If a doctor or healer is genuinely calm or kindly and shows friendliness and empathy in their first encounter and thereafter, they'll have a positive effect on the client regardless of anything they say, do, or prescribe.

If the doctor or healer strongly believes in themselves and what they do, their confidence will also be relayed non-verbally to the client or patient through facial expressions, breathing, and body language, and without doing anything they'll nudge the client toward adopting a positive belief about the forthcoming treatment.

This is partly why studies show that a positive or confident doctor tends to see better results in patients. It's also one of the reasons why much modern research, some of which I shared in the previous chapter, shows pronounced effects of doctor empathy. In this way, the state of a doctor or healer is an active ingredient and a very important part of *any* treatment, whether conventional or complementary.

Naturally, then, not all reiki healers will produce the same results, even if they perform identical treatments, just as not all doctors get the same results, even if they give identical prescriptions to people presenting with identical symptoms. This is one reason why the 21-day cleanse, a practice that newly trained reiki practitioners are asked to perform, is important. It helps them to *practice* being in a peaceful state while they work with reiki and to practice surrendering to the needs of their clients.

Repetitive Observation

The concept of emotional contagion, and also the idea that the MNS mirrors *any* movements, not only those of facial muscles, is now being used in sports and rehabilitation. In sports, several new studies have shown that learning a skill can be accelerated by 'action observation' – the repetitive observation of a correct action being performed.

Repetitive observation by a novice of a tennis serve or a golf swing performed by an expert, for example, can speed up learning of the serve or swing by stimulating the muscles in the same way as those of the expert, in effect 'wiring in' the movement more quickly than practice alone. Similarly, studies show that rehabilitation of stroke patients can be accelerated through the same kind of process – that of repetitive 'action observation' of an able-bodied person carrying out basic movements. It works in exactly the same way as emotional contagion.

2) Heart State Transference

The second way a reiki healer's state can affect a client is through the seeming contagiousness of their heart coherence. This may work alongside the MNS or it may be independent of it. To date, I'm not aware of any research that has examined the connection, although it seems to me that they're probably connected.

The HeartMath Institute has shown that when two people are in close proximity, the heart (and brain) of one person can entrain the heart and brain of the other, just as a large pendulum can entrain a smaller one. The healer has to be in a positive state for this to happen, because only then will their own heart rhythms be in a coherent state. Since a person's mental and emotional state impacts their heart coherence, their state can effectively impact that of the other person.

In a simple study to test this, volunteers were asked to hold hands. Within a short while, person B's EEG began to sync with person A's ECG. The brain waves of one person synchronized with the heart rhythms of the other. This was found in about 30 percent of people paired together for the experiment.[25]

In another study involving one hundred and forty-eight 10-minute trials, 15 trained 'senders' were asked either to focus on a feeling of care and compassion and direct it toward an untrained 'receiver' in close proximity, or to focus on their own heart coherence without trying to 'influence' the receiver.[26]

The researchers found that the receivers' heart coherence was affected by that of the senders'. Interestingly, the receivers achieved greatest heart coherence when the healer wasn't actually trying to influence them, but instead had focused on their own coherence practice. This is sometimes called the 'natural healer effect.'

Believing that healing is bi-directional – that is, it's affected by the relationship established between a healer and a patient – the researchers asked each person (healer and patient) how they felt about one another. It turned out that the strength of the entrainment was related to the strength of their emotional connection. This is consistent with research on empathy and emotional contagion, which are also stronger when two people have a closer emotional connection.

Reiki practitioners are trained to allow a feeling of 'universal love' to be their dominant state – a sense of love, empathy, compassion, and surrender to what is in the 'highest good' of their client. Through the agency of the MNS and heart coherence, their state almost certainly impacts on a client; and the strength of the effect is shaped by empathy, compassion, and any bond, however transient, that forms during the reiki session.

For more information on emotional contagion and how it works, see my book *The Contagious Power of Thinking* (Hay House).

Integrating Conventional and Complementary

The desire for and use of complementary medicine is increasing around the world. In many hospitals, reiki and other therapies are offered as a treatment alongside conventional medical care, and are certified by a doctor or nurse. Many conventional therapy practitioners work alone, however, in their private practices, which are outside of the sphere of our medical establishments.

Many doctors are afraid that endorsing complementary practices will result in some patients visiting a complementary practitioner instead of their physician; they worry that a person may be experiencing pain and that while the healing practice may alleviate it to a degree, it may in fact be a symptom of something much more serious that the complementary practitioner wouldn't be able to diagnose. As a result, by the time the patient seeks advice from their doctor, it may be too late to offer them the treatment they need.

For this reason, I'd like to see an officially acknowledged closer integration between complementary practitioners and conventional medicine. It's starting to happen already in the USA, UK, Europe, and around the world, as we discussed in the previous chapter and at the beginning of this one, but I'd like to see it broadening further.

Complementary therapy practitioners would need to receive some training so that they can swiftly refer a client to a medical doctor if they display any of the warning signs they've been instructed to look out for. If such a practitioner wishes to align with a medical board, they would be required to take a certification course with the medical board. In this way, doctors would also be able to refer a number of patients to complementary practitioners, if the patients are open to it.

Given the restorative and stress-reducing effects of reiki and other complementary practices, this might just be the tonic that a large number of patients need, and it could result in less need for the patient to return as frequently to their doctor, thus alleviating some of the burden on healthcare services worldwide.

CHAPTER 6

Crystals

Crystals and gemstones have fascinated humans for millennia. The Sumerians, creators of the world's earliest known civilization, located in the southernmost part of Mesopotamia (now southern Iraq), used these mineral rocks in their magical formulas.[1] In ancient Egypt, crystals and gemstones were embedded in jewelry and in talismans worn for healing and protection from evil. An amulet's power was determined by its color, size, and inscriptions, and also by the ritual that was performed with it. Wealthy Egyptians even buried their dead with a scarab carved from lapis lazuli, believing that it would protect their loved ones in the afterlife.[2]

The ancient Greeks are believed to have used crystals extensively too – in fact, the word crystal is derived from the Greek *krystallos*, which means ice.[3] In Europe during the Middle Ages, belief in the healing properties of crystals was widespread. Information about the stones and their perceived medical applications was collected in texts and books known as lapidaries.[4] And in North America, the Hopi Native American tribe have long used crystals to help diagnose illness, believing they can help a medicine man or woman to have clearer sight.[5]

Crystals enjoyed a huge popularity surge in the 1970s and 80s as part of the New Age movement, and more recently they've been at the forefront of the booming health and wellness craze, with people in their twenties and thirties making up a large portion of those who use, carry, or wear them.[6] Large commercial brands are adapting to this millennial market: 'mystic beauty' – which includes crystals in jewelry and spiritually themed beauty products infused with crystals – is a growing trend.[7]

This renewed enthusiasm for crystals among young people also has a spiritual component. Researchers at Scotland's University of Stirling reported that young people are selecting different spiritual and religious elements from the 'spiritual marketplace' and mixing them to form their own individual beliefs and practices, rather than tying themselves to a single belief system or practice. According to some research, this pick-and-mix spirituality is fueling some of the rise in popularity of crystals today.[8]

In this chapter, we'll look at some of the myriad ways in which crystals are used in the modern world, as well as how they work in meditation and healing practices.

Crystals and Technology

Quartz crystal is used abundantly in modern technology. Fifty years ago, a pendulum swing was used as the source of timekeeping vibrations, but today clocks and watches use quartz and rely on the piezoelectric effect, in which an electric current from a battery causes the crystal to vibrate exactly 32,768 times a second.[9]

Ultra pure natural quartz particles are used to produce the silicon for silicon chips, which are used in all computers and smartphones.

The Palomar Observatory in Southern California is the site of the Hale Telescope, one of the world's largest reflecting telescopes, the main mirror of which measures 16 feet 5 inches (5 meters), weighs 14.5 tons (20 tonnes) and was created by melting quartz at around 2,732°F (1,500°C). The telescope has led to immensely important discoveries about the nature and structure of the universe.[10]

Most of the grains of sand on any beach in the world are quartz. The windowpanes in your house and in your car also began as quartz particles that were melted and cooled. Optical fibers for phone and broadband start out as quartz too. It's melted at high temperatures and then quickly cooled to form a glass, which is pulled into fibers. These fibers have a property that allows total internal reflection, where light bounces off the insides of the fiber instead of shining out of it; this enables light to stay inside the fiber as it travels through it, making high-speed networks possible. In this sense, quartz is responsible for the superfast communications that take place daily all over the world.

Quartz is the main constituent of granite, too, making up between 20 and 60 percent of it. Many ancient buildings, including temples and the Great Pyramid at Giza in Egypt, are limestone and granite based.

Recrystallization

Benoit Mandelbrot, coiner of the word 'fractal,' wrote that quartz crystals form in highly fractal patterns. This means that if you were to cut up a piece of quartz into smaller and smaller fragments, these pieces would resemble the whole.

In fact, if you view any crystal using X-ray diffraction, a technique for looking at the structure of things at the atomic scale, you'll find that even at the level of just a handful of atoms, it resembles the tips of larger crystals. Using a technique called recrystallization we can coax lots of atomic-scale crystals together to form large crystals of a variety of substances that are often indistinguishable from the crystals on sale in a New Age store.

Many of the drugs we take when we're sick can be made to recrystallize into such a crystalline form. About 90 percent of all prescribed and over-the-counter drugs are actually composed of tiny crystals.[11] Drugs are not so practical in this form, though, as they need to be combined with other ingredients (excipients) to maximize their effectiveness.

About 65 percent of a typical adult's bone mass is crystal, too (a type known as hydroxyapatite.)[12] According to the National X-Ray Crystallography Service at Southampton University in the UK, even chocolate is crystal and has six crystalline forms. Chocolate's different forms, tastes, and textures come from different amounts of cocoa butter, which determines the type of crystal that chocolate forms. We even eat crystals every day in the form of the salt in our food.

Quartz Protection

Crystals are the most natural structures in our world; in fact, they're its building blocks. Quartz is made from silicon dioxide (SiO_2). It mostly crystalizes from molten magma and is the second most abundant mineral in the Earth's crust.

> **Quartz crystal is a protector and healer of the Earth.**

That might sound somewhat mystical, but recent research at the Tokyo Institute of Technology in Japan, published in the prestigious journal *Nature*, suggests that it's the formation of quartz crystals deep inside the Earth, close to the core, that powers the planet's magnetic field, also called the geomagnetic field (GMF).[13]

The GMF envelops the Earth and protects us from harmful cosmic rays. Life on Earth simply couldn't survive without it. And, regardless of opinions as to whether or not quartz crystals possess healing properties for humans, they certainly have healing properties for the Earth itself.

Earthquakes occur when the Earth's crust slips along a fault line, such as the Ring of Fire that stretches from New Zealand through the Philippines, up through East Asia and Japan, over to Alaska and down the west coast of Canada, the USA, and South America. The San Andreas Fault in California is one of the fault lines within the Ring of Fire. Publishing in *Nature*, scientists from the Department of Earth and Planetary Sciences at McGill University in Montreal, Canada, recently showed that following an earthquake, quartz crystals quickly begin to form along the fault line as the crust cools, binding the two sides of the 'cut' together, like internal sutures, and 'healing' the Earth's wound.[14]

Sensing the Earth's Magnetic Field

Many people use crystals in their garden because they believe they help plants to grow. Is this woo-woo, or might there be some valid reasoning behind it?

Quartz crystal is a diamagnetic substance, which means it repels the Earth's magnetic field (GMF). Quartz sends the GMF around itself a little, like the way an umbrella bends the path of rain as it falls around us. And just as our umbrella sends more rain onto someone standing beside us who doesn't have one, a diamagnetic substance essentially passes the GMF over, increasing how much is felt by something in the vicinity.

Plants are tuned to the GMF. The study of this phenomenon is known as plant magnetoreception, or sometimes magnetotropism. It's a relatively new field of science, in part motivated by understanding how plants will grow in space or on other planets, such as Mars, where they'll experience different magnetic field strengths.

Magnetoreception and Plant Growth

Hundreds of studies now show that experimentally increasing or decreasing the GMF has considerable effects on plant growth. It affects the germination rate of seeds, the uptake of water, shoot growth, photosynthesis, flowering time, and even biomass accumulation.[15]

The specific effects vary from species to species; some plants grow a little faster in a higher magnetic field strength and slower when the strength is reduced, yet other species grow slower in a stronger magnetic field and faster in a weaker one. It seems to depend on their genes.

Altering the Earth's magnetic field strength can even help plants make better use of available water, something especially important in dry environments. When scientists in the Department of Agricultural Physics at the ICAR-Indian Agricultural Research

Institute in India's New Delhi pre-exposed chickpea seeds to a weak magnetic field for one hour, there was a 60 percent increase in water uptake compared with seeds not treated with the magnetic field.[16]

Most of the studies expose seeds or plants to magnetic fields while they're growing, but in some studies, it's the water that's exposed to the magnetic field instead of the seed or plant. Yet the results are similar. In one study, weakly magnetized water increased the yield, chlorophyll content, and net rate of photosynthesis in plants.[17]

Diamagnetism and paramagnetism – aligned with a magnetic field rather than opposed to it – seem to affect plant growth, and in part this is due to effects on the GMF. Dia- and paramagnetic effects are smaller than the previous experimental studies, which involved making relatively large changes to the GMF, but the effects are currently being examined.

The research is at a very early stage and thus far is focused on the effects of diamagnetic metals that are present in soils, such as zinc. One 2020 study found that zinc affected the uptake of iron in plants by altering the expression of a gene for an enzyme that controls iron uptake.[18] The scientists reported that it was the diamagnetism of the zinc that was responsible for this and indicated that they were now studying diamagnetic and paramagnetic effects further to investigate the extent to which they affect plant growth.

The reason for these genetic effects seems to be that diamagnetism and paramagnetism induce small changes in magnetic fields. And even though the changes are relatively small, they seem to be important all the same. It seems to me that it's quite possible that small changes in the GMF in and around a plant caused by diamagnetic quartz might produce measurable effects in it, just as diamagnetic metals like zinc do.

Can Crystals Affect Plant Growth?

There's no formal research (that I'm aware of) that has studied the effect of quartz crystal on plant growth, but there have been several online reports of home experiments, some by experienced gardeners, some by amateur scientists, and others by children for school science fair experiments.

None of this research has been published in peer-reviewed journals, but that doesn't necessarily mean there's nothing of merit in it, only that we should keep our minds open to the possibility that the testing protocol is insufficient to prove anything or that the results could be flawed or wrongly interpreted. But in some science disciplines it's often the case that a rough observation is made which, on further and more detailed investigation, turns out to be true.

The peer-review process of publishing scientific studies is the best thing as it allows other researchers to spot any potential errors; and also, if the work is valid, either to replicate or develop experiments to further test a phenomenon. But it's not always an option; lay people don't publish for any number of reasons, especially when they're conducting inexpensive home experiments.

Experimenting with Rose Quartz Water

I did some experiments of my own that I've never published anywhere. My hunch was that the diamagnetic or paramagnetic properties of some crystals may have an effect on seed growth. I also wondered if the main effect, or at least part of it, would be via the water used to feed the plants.

My reasoning was based on my research as an organic chemist. In my work, I frequently used an analytical technique known as infrared spectrophotometry, which detects changes in chemical bonds as they stretch and vibrate and as molecules interact with each other.

I knew that subtle changes in the local environment of water could induce changes in the way the molecules arrange themselves through what's known as hydrogen bonding. It's the phenomenon that gives water the surface tension that allows the family of insects called *Gerridae*, otherwise known as pond skaters or water striders, to skate across its surface.

I wondered whether tiny changes in hydrogen bonding in water induced by the presence of a diamagnetic quartz crystal would translate to a change in the growth rate of seeds. I chose cress seeds for my experiment because they grow quickly, which means any change produced by the presence of a crystal would be easier to spot.

I split 300 seeds into six pots of 50 seeds and watered them once a day. I chipped a small piece off a large rose quartz crystal and partially crushed it into small splinters (in hindsight, this might have altered the properties of the crystal due to the piezoelectric effect). I then taped the splinters to the underside of a plastic cup and poured mineral water into the cup. This is the water I used to water the seeds.

The reason I placed the crystal splinters underneath the water and not in it was to avoid any possible contamination of the water by anything that was in the crystal. It was possible that some finely ground silica from the crystal could dissolve in the water, for instance. I made an assumption that the diamagnetism of the quartz would still impact the water, even though it wasn't directly in it.

I extracted 1 ml of water each day for seven days to water the seeds. I compared them with six pots of 50 seeds watered under the same conditions but using water without any crushed crystal underneath it.

The results were quite significant. After seven days of watering, the sprouts from seeds watered with the rose quartz water, as I called it, were about 30 percent taller than those watered with ordinary water. The difference was visible, but I measured each sprout by hand to be sure. Of course, there could have been errors in my experiment, which would have been spotted through peer review.

Despite my lack of controls and peer review, I've included my results in this chapter, in the event that it does reflect a real effect of some crystals on plant growth through their diamagnetic (or paramagnetic) properties, and perhaps to encourage readers to try out their own home experiments.

Other Informal Experiments

Other home experiments that have found their way online are worth a mention here. In one, different crystals were added to distilled water, which was then used to water plants; the result was growth rate increases in arugula (rocket) seeds and plants and sunflower seeds. The crystals used were amethyst, quartz, rose quartz, and green aventurine.

> **People have placed crystals directly in the
> soil and found that quartz had a significant
> effect on the growth of different plants.**

In another experiment, tomato plants grew visibly taller, were much more vibrant, had greener leaves, and produced larger, riper tomatoes in a faster time when compared with plants without crystals in the vicinity.

Neither my experiments nor any of the others mentioned earlier would stand up to peer review, as they weren't properly controlled. The tomato plants could have experienced different soil conditions or even have had more sunlight, for example. But this doesn't mean they don't have merit.

My assumption that the crystals might affect the hydrogen bonding in the water possibly has some validity. Research on the rate of crystallization of zinc sulfate, a substance that's often used in zinc dietary supplements, found that it changed in the presence of magnetic fields.[19] The researchers suggested that water had some 'magnetic memory' that it retains for up to 150 minutes. As I had, they assumed that the magnetic field altered the hydrogen bonding between individual H_2O molecules and suggested it's where the magnetic memory lay.

Water is a major component of both plants and our bodies (which are about 75 percent water), so minor changes in the GMF caused by diamagnetic and paramagnetic substances may affect water on that microscopic scale. The effect may be small, but it could be enough to produce important effects in fast-growing plants.

Magnetoreception in Humans and Animals

As amazing as it sounds, it appears that humans are tuned to the Earth's magnetic field too. Researchers at Caltech in California invited volunteers to sit in the dark on a wooden chair, facing north, in an electromagnetically shielded cage. Then they shifted the direction of a magnetic field equivalent in strength to the GMF.

The brains of the volunteers reacted instantly, even though they had no conscious awareness of any change. Alpha brain waves in the 8–13 Hz range changed, which is a range associated with sensory and cognitive processing, including the processing of sights, sounds, and touch.[20]

And the change in brain waves depended on which direction they shifted the magnetic field. People in the northern and southern hemispheres experience a different direction of field. The fact that the volunteers reacted only to a specific direction, wrote the Caltech researchers, showed that they were 'tuned' to the local GMF.

The researchers suggested this ability is likely due to the presence of magnetite crystals in specific brain cells. Magnetite crystals align with magnetic fields and are known to cause some bacteria (magnetotactic bacteria) and even some species of animals to be sensitive to the GMF.

Recent research published in the journal *Nature* has lent support to this finding. Researchers from the Department of Earth and Environmental Sciences at Ludwig-Maximilians University in Munich, Germany, mapped the presence of magnetite crystals in the human brain and found it spread throughout it, but with higher concentrations in the cerebellum and brain stem as well as elevated levels in the pineal gland.[21] These are ancient locations and hint that over eons, humans most likely did become tuned to the GMF, only we just don't consciously use it today.

The Avian Magnetic Compass

Magnetoreception is present in plants and humans, and it now appears to be fundamental in much of nature. It's been found to be widespread in birds, insects, and some marine animals. Some birds even have a photopigment in their retinas containing a molecule called cryptochrome that allows them to see the Earth's magnetic field as clearly as we might see a road with lines painted on it.[22]

The birds see a magnetic road, which is believed to appear augmented over the landscape, like virtual reality light structures lain over the world that we humans see. It helps them travel huge distances as they migrate for the winter, only to return in the spring, not only to the same town but also to the same branch of the same tree in the same garden that they left months earlier.

When scientists artificially shift magnetic north, many birds immediately and abruptly alter their heading in line with the new magnetic north, as if the 'road' had simply veered to the left or right. Birds even use the inclination, or dip angle, of the GMF to tell them how far north or south they are. Their magnetic compass is now known as the avian magnetic compass.

Marine animals have something similar. Loggerhead turtles use the direction of the GMF to travel huge distances to lay eggs. A tiny change in the GMF can alter a bird's heading or change the direction in which a whale, dolphin, or turtle is swimming. Even cattle tend to align themselves with the GMF.

So it shouldn't be so surprising that magnetoreception is innate in humans. It basically means that human biology reacts to changes in the GMF. The Caltech researchers proposed that even though human magnetoreception is now largely unconscious, the brain reacts all the same.

The question is, if small changes induced by diamagnetic or paramagnetic substances do impact on plants, could they impact on humans too? I think we certainly can't rule it out. How much it affects us, and whether particular brain and body locations and biological processes are more susceptible, no one yet knows.

Clear Quartz, Clear Mind

Over and above their possible diamagnetic and paramagnetic effects, humans are influenced by crystals in other ways. Dzogchen, or the Great Perfection, is a teaching in the Tibetan Buddhist tradition that aims to guide practitioners to discover the ultimate basis of existence – the nondual state of perfection. This basis, or ground as it's sometimes called, is believed to have qualities of emptiness (purity), luminous clarity, and compassion.

In the transmission of Dzogchen, teachers use a quartz crystal sphere to represent the perfect clarity of an individual's natural state. The quartz is said to symbolize the clarity of mind that one seeks and the purity of being that's one's essential nature.

Clear quartz is used in a similar way by people across the world who work with crystals; to them, the crystal's clarity represents the mental state they wish to attain and the natural state of being.

> *For some healers, the fact that quartz is formed deep within the Earth symbolizes inner stability and an ever-present connection with our deeper spiritual nature.*

Some people meditate while holding a quartz crystal, while others place the stones where they're visible, such as on an altar or a table. In these ways, and in Dzogchen, the crystal functions as what's known in cognitive psychology as a representation.

Essentially, a representation is one thing standing for (representing) another thing – in the way that a heart emoji represents love or the skull and crossbones symbol represents a toxin. In Dzogchen, the clarity of a quartz crystal represents the pure state of mind a person seeks to attain and thus helps them move toward it.

This is because representations and other symbols can and do affect our thinking, how we feel, and even our brain and body chemistry. For example, letters and words have no meaning of their own – they're merely symbols that represent things for us. But these symbols clearly impact our feelings and behavior, and for this reason, some cognitive psychologists refer to the mind as a symbol operating system.[23]

As an example, the cross stamped on an aspirin tablet manufactured by the German pharmaceutical company Bayer enhances its painkilling effect because of what the red cross symbol represents to us (rescue, relief, being saved by the International Red Cross).

The extra effect is driven by the production of endogenous opiates in the brain – a real chemical change that's due to what the symbol represents. Also, a mental representation of biting a slice of lemon can even make us salivate.

As we explored in Chapter 1, neuroscience has shown that mental representations (or visualization) can help accelerate the learning of new physical skills, and in studies this has helped novices improve in sports, experts deepen their talents, injured people recover faster, and stroke patients speed up their rehabilitation. A mental representation of the immune system doing its job can even aid the immune system.[24]

This is why quartz crystal can help us feel mentally clear and focused. The clarity, shape, and feel of the crystal *represents* the mental state we seek to attain. With extra clarity and focus, a person is better able to accomplish their work, whether spiritual or practical, or achieve their goals.

Amplifying Intention

Advocates of crystal healing use quartz in any situation where increased clarity or better focus is beneficial. Some believe it helps them become more still of mind or clearer during meditation or prayer. Others use it to communicate with spirit guides or deceased loved ones; to these people the clear crystal represents themselves as a clear channel to spirit communication. Putting aside for now any preconceptions about people's spiritual beliefs, it's clear why quartz and other crystals can be helpful in these ways.

It's sometimes claimed that crystals can be used to 'amplify intention.' This is another way of saying they can help to focus the mind and in so doing make an intention clearer and therefore stronger. As such, they increase our likelihood of achieving a goal.

I think that some of the discord that exists between crystal therapists (or reiki practitioners) and skeptics of these modalities comes down to a misunderstanding of each other's use of language. To most skeptics the idea of creating a greater mental focus that makes us more likely to achieve our goals is acceptable, but when this process is referred to as 'amplifying intention,' it sounds woo-woo.

Ultimately, the same message is being conveyed, but it's couched in different languages. Amplifying intention represents clearer, amplified focus, or even a clearer link with our spiritual essence, that helps us bring about the achievement of goals, whether practical or spiritual.

The Science of Association

Amplifying intention through the use of crystals can be thought of in another way too – using the science of association. Try the following. Pick up a stone, a small pebble or something similar. Now think of something important to you as you simultaneously squeeze the stone or turn it over in your hand. Do this for about five minutes and then lay the stone down.

Later in the day, pick up the stone again. You'll notice that you spontaneously recall the important thing you'd been thinking of when you first picked up the stone. Why? Because you created an *association* between the stone and the important thing you were thinking of. If the important thing was a goal, you'll find that having an association between that and the stone will help you to move toward it. Having the stone around will help you to maintain your focus on the goal.

> **Research shows that the more frequently we focus on a goal, the more likely we are to achieve it.**

You'll find that it will be most helpful to keep the stone somewhere you can see it throughout the day, such as on your desk or mantelpiece. You might even find it helpful to carry it in your purse, bag, or pocket.

There's a reason I'm speaking of a stone here and not a crystal. A lot of people are skeptical about using crystals in this way, and so to them, a stone feels more palatable. When I first described this process to others I referred to using a crystal instead of a stone; it was met with skepticism, despite the obvious way in which it works. When I reframed it with a stone in place of a crystal, it seemed to make more sense.

This is what I refer to as knee-jerk skepticism and it was one of my motivations for writing this book. People are skeptical of subjects not because they're experts in them and know what's true or not, but because they're *not* experts, and to them, the subject just doesn't *sound* plausible.

Speaking Different Languages

Crystal therapists and others who work with crystals sometimes call the process I described earlier 'programming' their crystals with a specific intention. It's another quirk of language that's frequently misunderstood by those skeptical of crystals. Some imagine their intention held as light (consciousness) in the crystal that's then transmitted outward into the universe, just as a crystal refracts light. The visualization process is the way they represent the use of the crystal in achieving their intention or goal.

How a person understands the way something works shouldn't be of concern; in many circumstances, the fact that it does seem to work is more important.

Science often focuses on the how and labels a practice pseudoscience if those who follow it interpret it in a way that differs from what science recognizes is going on, or if they use language that suggests they don't understand the science.

I often spend time in the company of people who describe certain practices using spiritual or metaphysical terminology, and although I'm a scientist, I understand what they mean because I've learned the 'language.' Once during a lecture I was attending, an apparently intellectual man in the audience verbally attacked the presenter, a young girl wearing a flowing dress and a flower in her ear, almost pushing her to tears as he took issue with the 'unscientific' statements she was making. She was entirely correct in what she was saying, but the man simply didn't understand her language.

Just because I may have formulated a scientific mechanism in my mind of *how* something works, it doesn't give me the right to minimize a person's practice by taking an intellectually superior position. And it also doesn't make me more right than them.

It shouldn't matter whether a person 'programs' their crystal and imagines a unicorn spirit flying out of it and spreading their intention like magic dust throughout the land, or whether they break it down into the science of association.

> *Visual imagery, even magical imagery,*
> *is simply a way to focus our attention on*
> *what we wish for or want to achieve.*

In fact, there's a great attraction in magical imagery because it's artistic and it resonates with our childhood dreams and our memories of the idea of a magical world, from a time when we believed that anything was possible: a belief that, quite frankly, many adults would benefit from today. I think some of us would do well to have a play with some magical imagery from time to time, even if it's just as a way to reduce stress.

People have a right to see the world how they wish. If someone wants to imagine a magical world, then it seems to me that in the interest of living in peace and harmony, we should celebrate it with them.

The Psychology of Color

A crystal's color can induce effects in us, too. Over and above a crystal's clarity or physical properties, its color is one of the reasons why people choose it for a particular purpose. We have inbuilt psychological associations with colors that have evolved over eons, such as the association of a blue sky with a state of calm.

These associations, studied in the science of color psychology, can elicit particular emotions and even influence our perceptions and behavior. Color associations are so ingrained that they even affect brain processes, and this is especially true when it comes to the flavor of foods.

In a study that compared the taste of M&M sweets, volunteers felt that the brown ones had a greater chocolatey flavor than the green ones, yet they contained exactly the same amount of chocolate.[25]

In another study, when a cherry-flavored drink was colored green, 37 percent of volunteers couldn't taste cherry at all and instead swore it was lemon or lime flavored.[26] The brain processed the taste in accordance with what the drink should be, given its color, rather than what it actually was. Similarly, in a study in which pineapple sherbet was colored pink, many volunteers couldn't taste pineapple.[27]

In pharmaceutical drug marketing, 'hot' colors like red and orange are preferred for stimulants because they induce stimulating effects. Sedatives, on the other hand, tend to be cooler colors, such as blue. In both cases, the color itself shapes the activity of the nervous system.[28] (You may remember the example I shared in Chapter 1, in which blue placebo sedatives were 2.5 times better than pink ones.)

Color can influence behavior too. One study that looked at the use of color in shop window displays found that the use of red tended to increase spontaneous purchases: in part this was due to its stimulating effect.[29] In Buchanan Street in the city of Glasgow, Scotland, the council installed blue street lighting in 2000 purely for aesthetic reasons, but surprisingly, rates of crime dropped substantially.[30]

While there may have been other factors that led to the reduction in crime, and it's difficult to pinpoint a single cause, it's quite likely that the blue lighting had an effect. Having walked that street many times myself, I can say that it does make it feel peaceful.

Marketers use color to influence a consumer's perception of a product and alter their likelihood of purchasing it. This is why bread is often sold in packaging that has brown or golden tones – the color promotes the sense of home baking.

Similarly, the British assorted chocolates Quality Street are packaged in a purple box because purple is associated with quality and royalty. Orange is a fun, lively, playful color that's effectively used by The Home Depot in the USA and B&Q in the UK, large chains that promote DIY, while the British low-cost airline easyJet uses the color to paint a picture of air travel that feels less businesslike and more about fun family holidays.

While lighter blues tend to be calming, darker blues can give the impression of competence and good communication; this has helped Facebook, although Mark Zuckerberg apparently chose blue for the company's logo because he is red-green color blind and blue stands out more for him.[31]

Starbucks' logo started out brown in 1971, representing the color of coffee, as well as the earthiness and ruggedness of the land on which it's grown; however, it changed to green as Starbucks grew, with that color being a representation of growth, naturalness, and eco-friendliness.

The important point is that the ingrained associations we have with colors impact us psychologically. They elicit real emotional effects; they can alter nervous system activity; and they even impact on brain processing.

The Color of Crystals

Some of the documented benefits of crystals are related to the effects of their colors, or are logical extensions of those benefits. Here are a few examples:

Pink

Rose quartz is said to help attract love; this makes sense because the color pink can help some women to feel more feminine and confident in themselves. Rose quartz is also believed to assist with a person's emotional healing; this may indeed work because pink is also a nurturing and soft color that's associated with the heart.

Blue

Turquoise crystal is believed to help a person feel more calm and balanced. Like the color of the sea off the coast of Sardinia, Mallorca, or Turkey, or throughout the Caribbean, the color of turquoise eases the human nervous system.

Lapis lazuli, a bright blue crystal, is associated with calm and harmony, but also with self-awareness, competence, and communication. These are all blue associations. For some, lapis lazuli also represents psychic protection. It's also the shade of blue used for Viagra tablets, which was no accident. A relaxed nervous system helps facilitate production of nitric oxide, which dilates the arteries, which is essentially what Viagra does. Similarly, blue elicits a sense of competence.

Red

Red jasper is associated with energy and vitality, which are qualities associated with the color red. The ancient Egyptians associated red jasper with the fertilizing blood of the god Isis, which may be why many crystal therapists today also associate it with fertility and rebirth.

Yellow

Citrine is a crystal said to help develop joy, success, and wonder, and help a person feel more enthusiastic. These are all qualities associated with the color yellow. Kyle Gray, the author of *Angel Prayers* and *Raise Your Vibration*, who teaches crystal therapy, refers to yellow citrine as 'the Sun in stone form.' Some crystal therapists even use yellow citrine to help attract money because the yellow qualities of joy and happiness elicit a positive state, which increases the likelihood of success in life.

Purple

Amethyst is believed to help us tap into our intuition. Purple is associated with quality and authenticity, which can be thought of as helping someone to feel more aligned with their authentic self and as a result, be more intuitive and less conflicted.

Green

Aventurine is believed to help us feel soothed and comforted, and these are properties associated with nature.

There are other claims for crystals that are more medical in nature, such as the belief that lapis lazuli helps boost the immune system, lower blood pressure, and reduce inflammation. There's no medical evidence I know of to support this, although these are the known physiological effects of being in a calmer state, which blue is known to induce.

Claims are also made for particular crystals – that such and such a stone will detox the liver, for example; I'm not sure how valid these are, and I'm a little reticent to attempt to validate them as I think if someone is in pain or has symptoms of illness or disease, they should first consult a doctor.

More Than Placebo

Skeptics of the use of crystals to promote well-being and facilitate healing sometimes point to a 2001 study presented by Chris French, Emeritus Professor of Psychology at Goldsmiths College at the University of London, who has conducted some scientific testing of paranormal beliefs and is former Editor-in-Chief of *The Skeptic* magazine.[32]

French asked the 80 participants to meditate for a few minutes while holding either a real quartz crystal or a fake crystal (which they were told was genuine). He also gave each person a booklet outlining 10 of the sensations they might experience, among them more focused attention, tingling, relaxation of the forehead, an improved sense of well-being, and activation of all levels of consciousness.

After meditating, the participants answered questions about whether they'd felt any effects from the crystal healing session, and it was found that there was no difference between the two groups. Seventy-four of the 80 participants experienced some of the suggested sensations, regardless of whether they'd held a real or a fake crystal.

It was a well-intentioned study, but as a writer and speaker on the placebo effect and the broader implications of the mind–body connection, I would have expected that result. Whether it was real or fake, each crystal was a *representation* of the effects listed in the booklet. The study wasn't necessarily a measure of whether or not crystals have effects – especially given the short time the volunteers held them – rather, it was more a demonstration of the power of suggestion. The volunteers experienced what they expected to happen.

The Crystal Bed

Our beliefs can *reduce* the effects of crystals too. Several years ago, while I was in Los Angeles, my friend Olivia took my partner and me to a shop that sold crystals. The owner escorted a few of us to a private room at the back of the shop and invited us to lie on a large blue 'crystal bed' – a hard crystal platform that was around 6 feet (2 meters) long and a few inches thick and made from a blue crystal that I believe was either angelite or lapis lazuli. She explained that in ancient times healers used beds such as this one, and that the understanding of their healing power has long been forgotten.

I lay on the crystal bed for about 10 minutes. I felt relaxed and experienced occasional tingling sensations; to me, it was therapy, just what I needed at the time. Next up was a man who was clearly a crystals skeptic. He lay on the bed for a few seconds before abruptly declaring: 'Nothing at all. It's just piece of rock and it's hurting my hip.'

He then spouted a few scientific facts and scoffed at the woman's claims that crystal beds had been used in antiquity – how could she possibly know, he insisted. One can't help wondering if his attitude hurt his hip more than the crystal bed did.

Both my experience and that of the skeptical man were valid. I chose to believe that there could be some truth in what the shop owner had told us, given what I knew about people's beliefs in the power of crystals. I opened up to the history and symbolism, and I decided to take her words on faith. I was curious. I wanted to believe. And as a result, I folded into the experience and it felt healing to me.

The skeptical man, however, had a different take, and his experience was in accordance with it. The dominant active ingredient for him was his attitude. It was stronger than the potential effects of the crystal bed – from its calming blue color and natural fractal patterns, to a resonance with the meaning and spirit behind the way ancient cultures may have used such healing tools. For both of us, attitudes and beliefs determined what we experienced.

As a science communicator I've learned that it's unwise for scientists to belittle people's beliefs just because they think they know more about the world and how things 'really' work. In the long term, scientists, and science, will fare better publicly if we employ more empathy and patience with people. Many people focus their intelligence in ways other than the academic; for example, most healers I know are high in both empathy and in emotional intelligence.

Crystals in Healing

Several years ago, I took a course in crystal therapy. I did so partly out of curiosity but also because, despite having spent seven years at university earning a science degree and a Ph.D. and then working in a technical environment in the pharmaceutical industry, I was feeling drawn to the seemingly softer and more holistic world of complementary medicine. I'd long had an interest in complementary practices and felt sure there was much to be gained by some kind of fusion of mainstream and complementary ideas within healthcare.

In the bi-monthly, year-long experiential course on which I enrolled, much of the focus was on using crystals as an aid to meditation, to help with focus, to heal emotions, and to attain higher levels of consciousness. We were taught about the uses and benefits of specific crystals and, in hindsight, much of this was consistent with Dzogchen and color psychology; for example, we learned that quartz crystal was for spiritual or mental clarity, which translated to higher consciousness.

A key practice was holding different crystals and noting how we felt. To me, blue crystals did indeed feel calming, while red ones were powerful, and yellow ones felt bright and cheery. The meditation practice helped us learn to draw on our intuition and to bring more conscious clarity to fleeting sensations and perceptions that the crystals elicited in us.

Naturally, each student was drawn to particular crystals in accordance with their own needs. I was drawn to an olive green crystal called moldavite. Unlike quartz crystals, which form in the Earth's core and make their way to the surface, moldavite isn't native to the Earth. It's a projectile rock, formed when a meteorite impacted the Earth around 15 million years ago. The teacher told us it came from the cosmos and represented the attainment of higher levels of consciousness.

At that time, higher consciousness – a sense of enlightenment that transcends everyday worries – was my goal, so I was drawn to moldavite because of what it meant to me. The teacher emphasized that it was how a particular crystal impacted on a person's consciousness – on their 'emotional energy' – that was all important.

Benefits of a Crystal Healing Session

I learned that crystals are tools that help facilitate mental, emotional, and spiritual shifts, especially if we meditate with them. To my mind, if there's a mental, emotional, or spiritual state correlated with a person's physical condition that the use of crystals has helped them to shift *away from*, then in some instances, some form of physical healing may possibly take place (as we discussed in Chapter 3).

Whether through the agency of color, or through beliefs about crystals, or about what they can help with, I could appreciate that crystals can assist in a person's emotional and physical healing.

I was taught that crystals can reduce stress, help balance our emotions, help us feel connected, increase the flow of energy in the body, and help dissolve emotional blockages. As part of the course, I offered crystal healing sessions to friends and family, who overwhelmingly reported feelings of deep relaxation and a significant easing of stress during the treatment; sometimes, they experienced powerful emotional releases.

If this is all a person gets from a crystal healing session, that's great. Because for a good many ailments it's exactly the tonic that people need. It's part of the attraction of taking a holiday or visiting a spa – the opportunity to let go of some of our tension and stress. If a crystal healing session can help with this, it's a positive thing.

As I mentioned earlier, I'd like to see complementary practices – including crystal healing – further integrated into mainstream healthcare, as there are a great many situations where a person might benefit more from a complementary treatment than a drug. But it would be safer if they were referred to a practitioner by their doctor.

Forming a Connection with a Crystal

Crystals, like drugs, have to be considered as part of a whole system of active ingredients, all working together – the person, the medicine (drugs, reiki, or crystals), the doctor, nurse, healer, or therapist, the environment, the sounds, and so on. In this way, there's a psychological entanglement between the person and the medicine, whether it's a painkiller, a person, or a crystal.

We must treat the medicine, the therapist, and the environment as a whole. We can't separate a thing from the person's consciousness *about* that thing – in a sense, they're a single object. Sometimes, the dominant effect comes from one side, sometimes from the other, but they're a single object nevertheless. It can be beneficial, therefore, to feel a connection with the crystals with which you choose to work.

> *Those who practice crystal healing take great care of their crystals – not only do they meditate with them and program them, but they also 'charge' them.*

I was taught to do this on the course, where it was suggested we use natural means. The purpose of charging a crystal is to help renew its association with nature and to cleanse it of any associations other than natural ones. It also helps give us the felt experience of caring for the crystal and, in so doing, deepen our sense of connection with it.

On the course, the best charging methods were considered to be placing the crystals outside during a full moon, or in natural running water, such as a stream. However, running them under a cold tap while saying a short prayer was also encouraged, or even performing what's known as 'sacred breath,' which is breathing gently onto the crystal while uttering the words 'I cleanse you with love.'

We were also advised only to handle our own crystals if we were going to use them for any purpose or for healing. I believe that the idea behind this was that the crystals would not then be associated with our impression of anyone who had handled them; if a crystal was handled by someone else, we were to cleanse it.

I found that treating my crystals in these ways helped me form a connection with them. They were more than just objects, they felt sacred – in the same way that one might revere a crucifix or other religious item. There was a definite sense of care that was born through this practice, and with hindsight, I believe that mattered greatly.

The Science of Crystal Healing

There's very little published research on the effects of crystals on humans. I think most academics would keep their distance from the subject, for fear of being associated with mystical practices. However, some independent holistic researchers have been a little more willing to study it.

Published in the *Journal of Natural and Ayurvedic Medicine* in 2018, one very small study conducted by a former chemistry professor at the University of Knoxville in Tennessee examined the use of crystals during reiki treatments.[33] She found that when the healer held a quartz crystal while giving a reiki treatment, the body's electromagnetic field was more coherent compared with when they didn't use a crystal.

In Chapter 5, I explained a little about how the electromagnetic field associated with a person's heart is modulated by their emotional state. This study wasn't designed to distinguish whether or not this coherence was due to any diamagnetic or paramagnetic effects from the crystal, or the effects of what the crystal represented in the psyche of the healer, or even from its color, but it could have been a general effect of using crystals in this way. Only further research will confirm this.

CHAPTER 7

How Perception Shapes Your Reality

In 2011, Vilayanur S. Ramachandran, a neuroscientist at the University of California at San Diego in the USA, published a paper called 'Colored halos around faces and emotion-evoked colors: a new form of synesthesia.'[1] It was the result of a study that he and his colleagues had made of a 23-year-old man with Asperger's syndrome (subject TK in the paper).

According to TK, as a child he'd had great difficulty understanding facial expressions and emotions (his own and other people's), and as a result he found it hard to interact socially. Aware of her son's struggles, TK's mother suggested that he attempt to match the feeling of an emotion (based on facial expressions) with a specific color, so he could relay the appropriate emotion to her and his father.

Pride became a light shade of blue, aggression was a red-pink, arrogance was purple, disgust was brown, compassion was orange, cheerfulness was green, love was pink, and so on. It's not clear whether TK came up with the color-emotion code himself or his mother did, or if it was born out of their own experiences and associations. Either way, the strategy helped TK immensely.

As he began to associate his own emotions with color and match colors with other people's facial expressions or how he felt about people, TK learned to 'read' others' emotions. And it wasn't just an intuitive reading – eventually, he began to see a halo, or aura, of color around people that betrayed their emotional state or how he felt about the person.

While you and I would get an intuitive sense of the way a person is feeling through emotional contagion, TK would literally 'see' their emotions. Despite some initial skepticism about whether the young man was really seeing this aura of color, Ramachandran and his team thoroughly tested him and confirmed that indeed he was.

Scientists had long viewed the idea of halos or auras – colors surrounding a living organism or creature – with enormous skepticism, but Ramachandran's research provided the first evidence of the existence of this effect. 'We demonstrate not only the authenticity of the phenomenon (that it is not made up by the subject) but that the colors evoked are perceptually real...' he wrote.

Synesthesia

Ramachandran and his team proposed that the color-processing region of the brain (known as V4) merged with the area for facial recognition (the fusiform face area) and areas involved in emotion, such as the amygdala, and empathy centers such as the insula. This merging, or linking up, is a form of synesthesia.

Synesthesia is a condition in which two or more regions of the brain that aren't usually connected are indeed connected. It allows those with the condition to smell color, for example, or see numbers as distances.

Of the various forms of synesthesia, the most common is grapheme-color synesthesia, in which letters and numbers are always perceived as colored, even when written in black ink on a white page. In spatial-sequence synesthesia, numbers are perceived as locations in space; for example, the year 1970 appears smaller or deeper in the page than the year 2021 because it's further away in time.

It's believed that approximately one in 23 people have some form of synesthesia and the condition is considered genetic. However, TK wasn't born this way – he'd effectively taught himself a means of perceiving and his brain had provided the necessary linkages through the natural process of neuroplasticity, which as we discussed earlier in the book is responsible for the brain changes that occur when a person practices meditation or visualization.

In the paper, Ramachandran raised the possibility that the emotion-color technique could be generalized. People around the world with autism (children and adults) could be taught it, and, in time, learn to *see* emotion and so better understand others.

Additionally, individuals who claim to see psychic auras have long reported that the colors they see show how a person is feeling. It may be that more people than we're aware of have learned something similar to TK, or even been born with this ability.

It's really just a form of intuition – one that takes on a visual element. Some people may indeed see intense colors around people and others may instead have an internal sensation of color. The human brain allows us to perceive in a multitude of different ways.

The Color of Reality

Do you find that when you're in a good mood the world appears brighter? And when you're sad, it seems grayer? Science now shows that sadness washes some of the color out of life, while joy brightens it. Happiness and cheerfulness make colors and textures seem more vibrant.

In one study conducted at the Albert Ludwig University of Freiburg, Germany, patients suffering with depression were asked to view a series of checkerboard patterns with varying degrees of black-and-white contrast. When compared to a healthy control group, the depressed patients were significantly less able to perceive the differences in contrast. The study suggests that depression can reduce color contrast, making the world seem monochrome and even flat.[2]

Sadness essentially impairs the richness of bright colors. Looking up at a blue sky while feeling sad washes out some of the brightness, leaving the blue a little grayer. It's why the world appears duller and less colorful when we feel down or depressed.

> *Our moods color our personal reality. When we're gloomy, the world reflects the way we feel. When we're happy, our world lights up with us.*

We create much more than grayness or brightness, though. Reality isn't at all what it appears to be when we look around us. As bizarre as it sounds, the world around you has no color at all until you add it; neither does your skin, hair, or nails. *You* create color in its entirety.

If you take a walk in a park and fix your attention on a patch of grass, assuming you're not color blind you'll note that it's green. But in that moment, you're creating *greenness* that doesn't exist in itself. And human skin isn't actually black, brown, red, yellow, or white: our eyes *create* the color.

Alien Worlds and Ultraviolet Vision

It's the cones – light-sensitive cells (photoreceptors) – in the retinas of our eyes that enable us to perceive color. Humans have about 7 million cones of three types. Dogs, on the other hand, have two types of cones. Humans have trichromatic vision – we see a broad range of colors and tones on the visible color spectrum – while dogs have dichromatic vision: they see only part of it; essentially, more cones means more colors.

Dogs, however, hear much higher frequencies of sound than humans do. We find it easier to accept this because it's common knowledge – we all know about those silent dog whistles with an ultrasonic tone that only dogs can hear – but the idea that we see differently to them too can sound a little woo-woo.

On a rainy day, dogs see a very different rainbow from us – an arc of dark blue, light blue, gray, light yellow, darker yellow, dark gray: a kind of blue, beige, gray-black. Our oranges and yellows are their brownish; our green is their beige.

Some species of fish, many birds, and insects are tetrachromats (four cones). We can't begin to imagine the alien landscape that they see – I say alien because it's completely invisible to us and if we suddenly developed an extra cone, we'd be unable to describe to our friends what we'd see.

Tetrachromatic vision even allows some of these species to see wavelengths in the ultraviolet range. Studies show that some birds use this for sexual selection.[3] Just as a human might have a preference for a partner with dark or light hair, these birds might choose a mate for the luminous, vibrating, effervescent 'colors' in its plumage, which to us look like regular feathers.

Many species of plants have diverse variations of color that extend well into the ultraviolet range. To you and me, they're just green, but they might be speckled with light and color to tetrachromats and surrounded by auras of colors that don't exist to us.

Pigeons and butterflies see an even stranger world. They are pentachromats, and for every color we see, they see 10,000 tones of it that are indistinguishable to us. As a result, their landscape is considerably richer than ours.

Who Perceives Correctly?

In reality, the world – everything around us – is more like a black-and-white movie than a color one. We add the color at the editing stage as our retinal cones grade the world for us. We see color because light bounces off an object, such as a blade of grass, the petal of a flower, or an orange, and its frequency is absorbed by the photoreceptors in our eyes.

Without these visual receptors, there is no color, only light and shade. Colors are therefore not properties of the objects themselves – they're qualities that we create, albeit without our conscious awareness.

So, does the human see grass more 'correctly' than a dog? Is the butterfly more 'correct' in its perception of a flower than us? We think of our eyes as cameras that take snapshots of reality, but they're not. No one sees actual reality. You just see your reality. Your perception shapes your experience.

As humans, we mostly see the same sort of picture, but that doesn't mean it's the true picture. If we underwent some fundamental change in the way our senses perceive things, then the world would suddenly appear alien to us. It would be the same world, but we'd perceive it differently.

Many neuroscientists and physicists believe that the 3D world we see is a shadow of something more fundamental, not unlike the shadows on the walls described in Plato's allegory of the cave. Each species, or perhaps each consciousness, *creates* 'reality' in a different way, forming the colors and textures – seemingly even the appearance of people and objects – around them.

Your Experience of Time

So, science has established that the human eye and brain together create the physical property of color, but what else do we create? What else doesn't exist on its own in the way we perceive it? It may surprise you to learn that we also create time, although in a different way.

In his 1890 book *The Principles of Psychology*, the American philosopher and psychologist William James wrote that 'the same space of time seems shorter as we grow older.'[4] His observation has now been verified by science. Our perception of the passage of time depends on how old we are, and time appears to speed up as we age.

For a child, the last few days before Christmas or another holiday feel like an age. But have you noticed that as you grow older, time seems to fly past all too quickly? Before long, the event you were excitedly anticipating is just a memory and it's accelerating away from you. You wish you could have held on to the experience just a little longer. This isn't just your imagination...

We really do experience time differently as we age. But we can speed it up or slow it down, just as we can see the world as brighter or grayer.

There are a few theories as to exactly how this works, so there's no real consensus, but it's a fact that we experience time speeding up as we get older.

One theory posits that the brain encodes novel experiences more than familiar ones, and that we therefore tend to remember new experiences more readily than those that have happened a hundred times. We easily forget monotonous things we've done repeatedly, but if something different happens just once, we tend to remember it. Taking the same route to work and having a job in which we do the same thing day in, day out actually accelerates time for us. Before we know it, we're in middle age and wondering where all the time went.[5]

Children encounter lots of new things, so time passes more slowly for them. However, when we reach adulthood time speeds up because we simply tend to have fewer new experiences. One way to slow time down as an adult is to engage in novel experiences. Examples include learning a new language, mastering a new dance, holidaying in a new area instead of the same place you always go. Even varying your route to work. Some neuroscientists now believe that novel experiences can help stave off Alzheimer's.

Your Perceived Lifespan

Another theory, first put forward by the French philosopher Paul Janet in 1897 that's only gaining more traction now because it might be simply a different way of looking at the earlier theory, is that as we age, a year becomes a smaller and smaller fraction of our whole life up to that point. Some call it 'log time' because time is compressed at the beginning but speeds up toward the end.

As an example, when you're 10, a year is 10 percent of your age at that point, and so it seems to last a long time. But a year to a 40-year-old is only 2.5 percent of their age, so it seems to pass four times quicker. A year to an 80-year-old passes even faster, about double the speed it did when they were 40.

I wonder how a newborn baby experiences time. The first few moments must feel like eons, because it's the entirety of their life at that point. They only know the present moment. In fact, the point at which human consciousness 'switches on' must feel like infinity. There is only now and it's completely new. In those first few moments after your birth, in fact, you've no perception of anything outside of yourself to attach labels and meaning to; while eons might pass in your experience, it only lasts a few minutes for your parents. Then, over the next few years, your parents experience you growing up much more quickly than it feels to you.

This is psychological experience, of course, but it's real all the same. Time is relative, and not just psychologically relative. Seemingly even more bizarre, time physically moves at different speeds, too.

Relativity

Time passes at different rates according to the 'shape' of space, which actually bends for different reasons. Our clocks and watches more or less agree, though, because the Earth is in a place in the universe where the shape of space is pretty uniform. But gravity bends space. We don't notice it because we all more or less feel the same gravity on Earth. But if you were out in space, you wouldn't feel the Earth's gravity and, as outlandish as it sounds, your watch would run a wee bit faster.

And it's not just your watch – it's time itself that runs faster. GPS satellites have to account for this; if they didn't, Apple Maps and Google Maps would be out by around 6 miles (10 kilometers) a day, and the satnav and other location services on your phone would be useless within a few hours.

And if you were near the edge of a black hole and subject to its super-strong gravity, your time would stretch like spaghetti. If you put out your arm, pointing it away from the black hole, it would age 100 years in the blink of an eye (an effect featured in the movie *Interstellar*, where a few hours on the surface of a planet close to a black hole was equivalent to 20 years on Earth).

But these are extreme conditions in space. On Earth, time runs at the same speed for all of us. Well, just about...

> *As strange as it sounds, in our homes time passes more quickly upstairs than it does downstairs, although the difference is imperceptible to us.*

Over a typical lifetime of about 80–100 years, living on the first floor of a house will age you about a thousandth of a microsecond more than living on the ground floor. In the same way, your head ages faster than your feet. Not much to fight over when it comes to who gets the top bunk, but it's true all the same.

So, just as there's no *true* color, there's actually no *true* time that's the *right* time, in the sense that there's not a single correct rate that time flows, nor a single experience of time that's more right than another. In the same way, there's no *true* space, no right measure of distance or the size of something.

Ultimately, there's no true reality. Time, space, color, even form are entangled with our perception and conscious experience of them. Reality is inseparable from our perception of it. It's impossible, in fact, to study *actual* reality, if there is such a thing, because our perceptions prevent us from getting to it. That's the message of the interface theory of perception.

Your Interface with Reality

As I sit typing these words, I pause for a moment and extend my hand to pick up a cup of coffee, which sits to the right of my laptop. How much of what I'm seeing is perception? Is it just the color of the cup? Is it the speed that my hand moves, or the time it takes for it to reach the cup? Or am I perceiving a distance between my hand and the cup that isn't actually true?

The interface theory of perception, created by Donald Hoffman, Professor of Cognitive Science at the University of California at Irvine, would say it's all perception.[6] There's no hand. There's no cup. There's no spoon. There's something, but the appearance of a hand and a cup are created by my brain.

Using computer programs running evolutionary simulations, Hoffman has suggested that reality is too complex for us to perceive it as it is, so our brain dumbs it down for us. He draws an analogy with a desktop interface on a computer screen. If you write, say, a letter or a dissertation on your computer and save it to your desktop, it appears as a colored icon on the screen. The icon isn't your actual work, but a representation of it.

A game on a computer or a smartphone is similar. The computer or phone screen is your interface. You can interact easily with the game and move your character left and right because you don't need to concern yourself with voltages and binary code. That's the computer's *reality*. Apps and games displayed on the screen simplify the computer's reality for you and allow you to interact with the game.

So there are two realities playing out at the same time – there's the computer's reality of voltages and miles upon miles of binary code, and there's your reality of a character moving across a screen. Which is simpler and easier to live with? The interface theory of perception says the brain always shows us the easy way. Space-time is our desktop. Everyday objects, mountains, trees, humans, animals, hands, and coffee cups, even the brain and its neurons, are icons, or representations, on our 3D screens.

So, when I extend my hand to pick up my coffee cup, there's a movement of something toward something else, but the hand, the cup, the physical act and what it looks like, even the notion of coffee and its flavor, is my perception.

We all agree that it's a hand, though, and coffee. But that's because we're of the same species and we've evolved in the same way from the same organisms over billions of years, and we occupy the same region of space in the universe that's subject to a seemingly steady passage of time. So our perceptions, not only of color and time, have evolved to be more or less the same.

Reality Is Symbolic

The interface theory of perception posits that reality is symbolic. Objects and events in our lives are symbols, like the subroutines of computer code that run in response to our perceptions and beliefs.

> **We don't see reality as it is, but as we are – as a representation of our conscious and unconscious states and beliefs.**

The theory hints that our consciousness paints the landscapes and scenery of reality, and even scripts the events and circumstances that occur on it; that our reality is a symbolic representation of the contents of our consciousness..

The idea that our consciousness can create our reality is a polarizing topic. Some say, of course, that we do create our reality. It's a given.

To others, it's the most woo-woo of all the woo-woo ideas and is declared as such with passion and the seeming authority of a fact. But it's not a fact – it might just be a belief.

It might be that we have more ability than we generally assume to affect meaningful changes in our lives – by influencing or even changing some of our symbols. That is, by changing the way we think about things, the assumptions we make, and the beliefs we hold about life and each other.

Hoffman has pondered this at length. In response to the question 'Knowing that reality is one of the symbols in an interface, can we manipulate reality with our consciousness?' he wrote: 'I'd say we're doing it all the time. We're so conditioned to believe that what we see is hard reality that the strength of this belief prevents us from seemingly changing reality. But the reality is that we're changing it all the time, but in a way that fits with our belief, hence we tend to not notice, or interpret the experience as chance or normal.'[7]

At the risk of over-speculating, I wonder if our deepest unconscious beliefs, like Jung's archetypes, are ones we collectively share and they govern the general rules about reality that humans experience: that fire burns and that solid objects are solid objects.

These are givens that we've experienced to be true since our earliest moments. They're core human symbols – the core subroutines of the operating system of human reality. But might a person alter some of these deep symbols, like hacking into the deepest layers of a code and making changes to the operating rules of a reality program?

Perhaps some of the miracles reported in some religious texts are true, or at least have a basis in truth. I've wondered if the foundation stories upon which superhero stories are written are based on unconscious beliefs about our true relationship with reality and its probable malleability at the hands of our consciousness.

I'm not suggesting that it's easy to access and alter these symbols of our metaphorical operating system, lest there be superheroes flying around us, but perhaps the odd person here and there has, either consciously or accidentally, bent a little of what we consider to be the general rules of reality.

While I was speaking about this once, someone remarked, 'If this is all true, then reality is just an illusion. I can pretty much do what I like. Nothing actually matters.' But this isn't the case. Regardless of how we perceive reality, we share it with each other. What we say and do *does* matter.

Regardless of how reality is perceived, we do perceive it in a human way. Regardless of perception, reality is clearly 'real' for us. We live in a shared world. We have communities and ultimately, we share resources, so we must live and work within a set of shared guidelines for peaceful and harmonious living.

Regardless of our relationship with reality, we should treat each other with kindness and respect. We shouldn't cause harm to anyone. We'd do well to show empathy and compassion and recognize that we're family. Maybe kindness is the symbol we should focus on the most in our world.

Chapter 8

Consciousness

In 2001, I undertook a trek in Peru with a group led by Stephen Mulhearn of Lendrick Lodge, who I mentioned earlier in the book. Among our experiences was a shamanic ceremony in the mountains. Under the supervision of Peruvian shamans, we consumed ayahuasca, a psychoactive beverage formed by brewing a number of plant roots and extracts native to the Amazon and used in ceremonies to assist in vision quests. Its active chemical ingredient is N, N-dimethyltryptamine, a substance with a similar chemical shape to serotonin (a neurotransmitter that we generally associate with mood).

Shortly after consuming the ayahuasca I looked up at the night sky and felt a shift in my perception. The stars began to warp and elongate. Soon I could read the sky as if it were a page of a giant book, although it wasn't in a language I would understand now.

It said: 'There is nothing outside of you. The whole world is a projection of your thoughts, feelings, loves, fears, hopes, and dreams. The fabric of the universe is love and it flows with intention. You need no special tools or techniques to heal or to create. All you need to do is believe.'

Fortunately, I had a notebook and pen in my rucksack, so I wrote down the English translation of the 'manuscript in the sky,' as I later jokingly called it.

Was this real? Was it a creation of my unconscious mind? Or is reality some kind of projection of consciousness? Or all of these? My experience seemed somewhat consistent with the view of the interface theory of perception, or the philosophy of idealism, which asserts that reality is indistinguishable from our perceptions of it, or the Eastern mystical view of nonduality (more on this later).

However, in the mainstream of science we tend to follow the philosophy of materialism – not because it's been proven to be correct, but because it works for most practical purposes – and the materialist view is that consciousness is a product of the interactions between neurons in the brain.

> *But could it be that consciousness isn't inside the brain at all, but everywhere in the physical world?*

Admittedly, this does sound a bit out-there. After all, we've had a lifetime of experiencing the sensation of, say, touching our arm and feeling it there. We've come to accept that 'I' am in this body. However, as unlikely as it sounds, this idea has enjoyed some serious consideration. It has a strong philosophical grounding and there's also strong scientific evidence in support of it.

The Hard Problem

If you fall and twist your ankle, you feel pain. That's your overwhelming experience. The next few moments for you are dominated by the feeling of pain. It can come in waves, or sometimes it's acute and goes away. Other times, it's a dull and persistent ache. But pain is your first-person conscious experience.

But your first-person conscious experience creates quite a problem in science. It's the essence of the 'hard problem of consciousness,' a term coined by David Chalmers, a professor of philosophy and neural science at New York University and co-director of the Center for Mind, Brain, and Consciousness. While the philosophy of materialism asserts that consciousness is created by the brain, the hard problem is about how and why we have first-person experience. How is it that I know myself as 'I'? And how is it possible that this first-person experience can arise from physical brain matter?

From a materialist perspective, pain is described as the transmission of signals along bundles of nerve fibers that then activate specific brain centers. But this view only tells us what the brain and body is doing while we have our pain experience. It's not the same as having the actual *felt experience* of pain. This is why many people are now beginning to question materialism.

Materialism is such a widespread assumption, though, and beyond academic philosophy, it's written about and taught as fact. So much so that any idea to the contrary tends to be considered nonsense. However, despite the assumption that most of us make to that effect, the matter is far from settled.

Philosophers and scientists hold many quite different ideas about what consciousness is and from where it arises.

While some materialists say that consciousness can be explained by processes in the brain, others say it's an illusion altogether. Dualists, on the other hand, believe that physical matter and consciousness both exist but that they're separate entities, like the idea of a body and a separate soul. Descartes was the most famous of the dualists.

Idealists say that consciousness is all there is, and that life and all things are simply how consciousness appears to us. Panpsychists, meanwhile, believe that all matter, even atoms and particles, has some form of conscious experience. Plato and Spinoza had panpsychist views.

The 'nonsense' label given to any alternative takes on the theory of consciousness – that it's not locked inside the head and that two or more people may therefore be connected, say, or that we might share subtle connections with nature, or even that our compassionate prayers for each other could sometimes help – isn't based on proof that these things are false, but rather, on our assumption that materialism is true.

While mainstream science has historically aligned with a materialist view, many scientists would call themselves dualists, particularly those with religious or spiritual views, and many are panpsychists or idealists.

However, if you ask a scientist their opinion on the theory of consciousness, most will say they tend not to think about it all that much, because it doesn't seem to matter in their field. If pressed, most will typically say that consciousness emerges from the brain, because that's 'just what seems to be generally accepted.'

Galileo's Big Mistake

But the accepted view of consciousness might not necessarily be correct, according to a number of academic philosophers and researchers in some fields of science. Philip Goff, Associate Professor in the Department of Philosophy at Durham University, UK, is one of them. In his book *Galileo's Error*, he argues that the hard problem of consciousness arises from the way we do science.[1] He traces this back to Galileo (1564–1642), the Italian astronomer, physicist, and engineer who is regarded as the father of modern physics.

Galileo established mathematics as the official 'language' of science. But the problem with this, according to Goff, is that while math is great at helping us understand how things work and how they interact, it doesn't tell us anything about what things actually are. That doesn't sound like much of an issue, but it leads us to our modern conundrum: neuroscience can tell us what the brain is *doing* when we have a conscious experience, but it can't tell us what the experience is actually *like*, what it *is*. There may well be much more to consciousness than we think, and it might have huge implications for life.

The problem is captured in the book *The Nature of Reality*, published by *New Scientist*, in which Sir Roger Penrose, Nobel Laureate in Physics and Emeritus Fellow at the University of

Oxford asks, 'What substance does this reality that we see about us actually have?'[2]

If we look inside our cells, to the DNA and enzymes, to the atoms that they're made of, and then peer inside the atoms themselves, we enter the domain of quantum mechanics. Here, we find particles such as electrons, protons, and neutrons, the latter two of which are composed of quarks, which are held together by gluons. Mathematics tells us that three quarks are bound together by gluons to make a proton, but it says nothing about what a quark or gluon actually *is* in itself.

Penrose concludes that 'the best we can do at this stage is refer to the mathematical equations that they satisfy,' and that what these things actually are 'is a notion that can only be understood in terms of the mathematics used to describe them.'[3] Part of what it leads to is that we can't measure consciousness in the way we conduct physical science, nor have we ever sought to.

> *Science is objective, while consciousness is subjective.*

If particles were people, it would be like only being able to talk about a relationship between them in terms of what they do, what happens when they come together – whether they hold hands or stand apart, or how long they're in each other's company – and not to acknowledge at all that they have identities and experiences and loves and fears, hopes and dreams.

We'd therefore describe their relationship in mechanical terms, with numbers corresponding to the directions in which they move; however, in so doing we'd have to ignore the experiential part. Yet the experiential part is what we know. It's what makes us human.

Goff writes that Galileo's error meant that science from his time onward would only ever tell us what things *do* but not what they *are*, which is fair enough because this aspect of science has allowed us to get to where we are as a society in the modern world. However, it does leave us with the hard problem of consciousness.

Why Does Solving the Hard Problem Matter?

A more complete understanding of consciousness and why we have first-person experience might lead us to a deeper understanding of mental health, and of how we interact with one other and form relationships, and even how we can live more harmoniously with each other and nature on our planet. It might lead to a deeper understanding of life itself. It may even answer the age-old questions: Who am I? Why am I here? What is the meaning of life?

It's really quite an important problem to solve, then, but outside of academic philosophy, it's generally swept under the carpet as we cling to a materialist view because it works for most practical purposes – even if it may well be wrong.

The Panpsychist Perspective

Panpsychists such as Philip Goff and his predecessors have attempted to solve the hard problem by proposing that rather than consciousness being produced by the brain, perhaps all of the matter that makes up the brain – even down to the atoms and particles themselves – has experience. Consciousness may be the intrinsic nature of matter. In a sense, quarks and electrons have soul – those that make up your body, those in nature around you, and those in the air you breathe.

To be clear, they aren't suggesting that a quark or an electron feels happy or sad, enjoys the sunshine, or likes to watch Netflix on a Friday night; as basic particles, their experience is basic too. But the combination of trillions and trillions of particles, each with its own basic experience, into something more complex creates our first-person conscious experience.

To panpsychists, more complexity is associated with more consciousness. It also means that everything, therefore, has conscious experience in one way or another. Not only are humans conscious, but animals, fish, birds, and insects are too. Trees, plants, and flowers also, therefore, have experience, as do rocks, crystals, mountains, planets, and the whole universe itself, because they're all composed of particles that each have experience – even if their experiences are vastly different from our own.

Panpsychists have their own hard problem, though. It concerns how particles of experience combine to give rise to the type of conscious experience that you and I have. But they believe that theirs is a much easier hard problem to solve.

At this stage, I'd like to point out that I'm not a philosopher. Many philosophers, mystics, Buddhist scholars, and others have dedicated their lives to gaining a deeper understanding of the world. There's much more to the philosophical views that I've described so far, but in the interest of keeping things as simple and lucid as possible, I've greatly condensed the ideas.

If you wish to know more about panpsychism, I'd recommend *Galileo's Error* by Philip Goff; if you'd like to explore the nature of consciousness and the hard problem, *The Conscious Mind* by David Chalmers is a good choice. If you're interested in a Buddhist fusion of science, spirituality, and consciousness, try *The Universe in a Single Atom* by His Holiness the Dalai Lama.

A Philosophical Conundrum

Avoiding either of these hard problems is idealism. In his paper 'Idealism and the Mind–Body Problem,' David Chalmers writes, 'When I was in graduate school, I recall hearing "One starts as a materialist, then one becomes a dualist, then a panpsychist, and one ends up as an idealist."'[4]

He expands on this by explaining that students of philosophy start out being impressed by science and its accomplishments, its medical advances and technological achievements, and so they come to believe that everything is made of particles of matter (materialism). But, as Chalmers explains, they soon encounter the hard problem of consciousness and come to realize that matter can't explain consciousness.

At this point, they become dualists, and believe that matter and consciousness both exist and are both fundamental things. But then, he explains, philosophers realize that physics only describes the structure of matter – what it does, but not what it is – and that it doesn't answer anything about its intrinsic nature.

They then play around with the idea that maybe the underlying nature of matter is consciousness itself, so they become panpsychists. But eventually, philosophers come to believe that consciousness is actually all there is, and that matter is just a *form* of consciousness, so they become idealists.[5]

Idealism and the Single Unified Consciousness

To idealists, consciousness is all there is. It's not created by matter, nor is it an experience of matter. All the different forms of matter – people, animals, nature, the universe – are just different ways that we experience consciousness, or more correctly, how we experience ourselves.

Consciousness is a unified whole. In an ocean, each wave seems individual – each might even experience itself to be individual – but it's part of the whole ocean. The wave rises out of the ocean and eventually, at the end of its lifecycle, it falls back into it again. Everything that we know is simply a *part of* the whole.

> *To idealists, we're like waves in an ocean, rising out of the whole, having a human experience, and eventually returning to it again.*

People, animals, plants, trees, mountains, crystals are different types of waves, different ways that the whole of consciousness appears.

Matter isn't something separate from consciousness, then, as materialists and dualists believe: matter *is* consciousness. The vast number of variations in different forms of matter and life are variations in the different ways that consciousness can appear. Like the different ways that white light can appear when it shines through a raindrop; you only have to look into the sky after rainfall to see white light show itself as red, orange, yellow, green, blue, indigo, and violet.

At least three Nobel Prize-winning physicists of the 20th century had views close to idealism. Louis de Broglie wrote, 'I regard consciousness and matter as different aspects of one and the same thing.' Max Planck, considered the father of quantum mechanics, said, 'I regard consciousness as fundamental.' And Erwin Schrödinger, one of the most famous quantum physicists of all time, said that 'the material universe and consciousness are made out of the same stuff.'

The interface theory of perception that we explored in the previous chapter shares a number of similarities with idealism, although its creator, Donald Hoffman, has referred to interface theory as conscious realism. Some philosophers regard them as very similar, though, differing only in some of the finer points.

Nonduality and the Illusion of Separation

Idealism is consistent with the Indian Vedic philosophy that we know of as nonduality. Reality – you and me, nature, the universe – is nondual. It's not mind (consciousness) and matter separately, but one thing appearing in two forms.

Clearly, we experience ourselves as being separate from one another. There's no denying what you see with your own eyes – that you and I are not the same person. But to idealists, this separation is an appearance only, like the separate colors of the rainbow that emanate from the same light, or the separate waves that rise and fall in the same ocean. Red and blue light in a rainbow might experience themselves as separate colors, but they're really different aspects of the same light.

In his book *I Am That*, the Indian sage Sri Nisargadatta Maharaj said that 'All separation, every kind of estrangement and alienation, is false. All is one.'[6]

Modern academic proponents of idealism are attempting to integrate it with modern science and bring the idea more to the fore in the West. In an outline put forth in *The Idea of the World* by Bernardo Kastrup, who has Ph.D.s in philosophy and computer engineering and previously worked at CERN, consciousness is described as an 'ontological primitive' – a philosophical term meaning that consciousness is primary, it comes first; that is, it's the basis of reality.[7]

Kastrup refers to each of us as 'dissociated alters' of the whole, in a similar way that a person with dissociative identity disorder can have multiple distinct personalities. We're individual personality units of the whole, like the colors of a rainbow, like waves on the ocean, billions of which appear over the planet at the same time. The whole is infinite, single, unified, unbounded consciousness. Humans, animals, plants, rocks, mountains, and clouds are separate only in appearance.

Some believe that the 'hard problem' for idealism concerns the way consciousness creates (or *seems* to create) matter. To imagine that consciousness creates matter though is to think from a dualist perspective – as if matter is separate from consciousness, a creation of it. But to idealists, matter is an *appearance* of consciousness – different symbols *within* it, not a creation *of* it.

In a sense, reality itself is a sort of symbolic projection of consciousness, in that it's how consciousness appears as the landscape of our lives and the forms and events that occur upon it. Many idealists and those who align with nonduality think of life as a kind of cinematic projection on a 3D screen that we call reality – but that the reel contains the contents out of our minds, even if these contents often feel hidden from us.

Kastrup writes, 'I am an idealist; that is, I subscribe to the notion that reality – despite being solid and continuous – is a projection of the mind.'[8] The physical universe 'out there' isn't out there at all, then, in the sense that it's separate from you. Despite appearances, you're entangled with each and every aspect of it – with every raindrop, with every grain of sand, with every leaf on every tree, with every person, with every cloud, with the oceans, with every planet, star, and galaxy. You and the universe are one and the same, simply different colors on the spectrum of consciousness.

I Am

Bhagavan Sri Ramana Maharshi, considered by many to have been the greatest Indian sage of the 20th century, said, 'As soon as one ceases to imagine that one is an individual person, inhabiting a particular body, the whole superstructure of wrong ideas collapses and is replaced by a conscious and permanent awareness of the real Self.'[9]

This 'real self' is the universe itself, the single unified consciousness. The experience of it is the goal of many advanced meditation practices. You are the universe, even if you don't feel it. While to materialists death is the end of life, to idealists there is no death, only the experience of a dissolution into the whole, like a wave returning to the ocean.

This view is somewhat compatible with those of the many people who have reported near-death experiences, or NDEs, even though these are widely viewed with skepticism. In her book *Dying to Be Me*, Anita Moorjani describes what happened as her body approached the end of its fight with stage 4 lymphoma.[10]

The attending doctors had told Anita's family that her organs were failing and that she was now in the final moments of her life. As she lay on a bed in a coma, her body riddled with a large number of tumors – many of them the size of lemons – at the base of her skull, all around her neck, under her arms, breasts, and abdomen, Anita experienced expanding to become the whole universe as an infinite state of unbounded consciousness.

As I sat with Anita and her husband, Danny, one evening in Glasgow, Scotland, after we'd both spoken at a conference there, I asked her what it was like. The only words that can adequately describe it, she told me, are 'I Am.' It was an infinity of experience, a one ness with all things, she explained. To add anything to those two words would make the infinity seem smaller. This type of experience has been shared by thousands of people who have had NDEs.

Anita said that she met her father and her best friend in the 'other realm,' as she calls it, and that their consciousnesses had dissolved into the whole. They told her that she needed to go back and 'live her life fearlessly.' She understood that was her purpose from that moment on, and that if she lived her life fearlessly, with absolute conviction and joy, to love and be kind, to respect herself and others, she would be free of cancer. Anita woke up from her coma, and days later, her tumors had shrunk by 70 percent; within five weeks she was cancer-free. Perhaps her experience was so profound that she'd hacked into the deeper symbols in the operating system of her reality.

A Law of Consciousness

David Chalmers wrote that consciousness must be natural and that therefore there must be natural laws that describe it. As we've discussed, there's no consensus on what consciousness is or where it comes from.

In the next chapter I present studies that look at the seeming connections between people regardless of how far apart they are (including telepathy). Studies of this type tend to be dismissed as pseudoscience, largely on the basis that they simply must be if consciousness is created by neurons in the brain. But if consciousness isn't locked inside our heads, as panpsychists and idealists propose, then such phenomena may have a scientific basis after all.

Before we get to those studies, though, and in the interests of attempting an explanation as to how and why they may be revealing something very important about reality, I'm free to speculate here. To begin with, let's suppose that matter is an appearance of consciousness. Let's run with that idea and see where it takes us.

If this is the case, then the physical laws we know about in life – those that govern movement, space, and time – must be appearances of consciousness too. So there might be some similarity between the way some physical laws work and how 'laws' of consciousness work. If a physical law tells us how physical things interact, then there might be a similar law about consciousness that tells us how consciousnesses interact.

Physical laws are usually written in the language of mathematics as equations. We've discussed Galileo's error, and so I think that if we want to show any links between the physical world and consciousness, we have to meet somewhere in the middle and talk about consciousness using the language of mathematics – not so much describing *what something is*, but *how things connect* with each other.

Thus, we have to take a mathematical equation that tells us how things in the world interact and see if a similar equation can tell us about what happens when two consciousnesses interact.

A Little Translation

Before we begin, please don't be deterred by the words 'math' and 'equation.' I'm not going to ask you to do long division and I'm not going to talk about 'x's and 'y's. If you'd prefer to skip this section, though, please go ahead. All you really need to know in preparation for the next chapter is that emotional connection matters... quite a lot. I've simply created a wee sentence in the language of math to show *why*. However, if you want to see how we can arrive at an equation for the interaction between the consciousnesses of two people, read on.

Many people assume that math is complex, but for most everyday purposes, it's quite straightforward. However, math uses a form of language that can put some of us off, so let me have a go at breaking that down.

Let's start with an example. If I have an apple and an orange, would you agree that I have two pieces of fruit? If I write that as a mathematical equation, it's $f = a + o$. It might seem more complex than a sentence in English, or whatever language you use, but it's just the math way of saying that the total amount of **f**(ruit) is made up of an **a**(pple) and an **o**(range).

The '+' sign represents the word 'and.' For ease, those who speak math shorten a word to its first letter – so here that's 'a' instead of apple, 'o' instead of orange, and 'f' instead of fruit. It keeps their sentences (equations) short and neat.

Einstein's famous equation $E = mc^2$ isn't so much different from our fruit equation. E is for energy and m is for **m**ass – the amount of something. It tells us that the energy in our fruit is related to the amount of fruit we have. So, if we had a bag of apples and a bag of oranges, then the amount of energy in our fruit is related to the mass of what's in those bags. The 'c^2' (c squared) bit is the speed of light squared, which I'll explain in a moment.

Rather than writing it in English, which would be 'Energy is equal to mass times the speed of light squared,' it takes up much less space on the page as an equation. It's the same thing, expressed in two different ways.

So, what about the c^2 bit – the speed of light squared? Einstein chose 'c' for the speed of light – it comes from the Latin *celeritas*, meaning speed. It's an exchange rate, like the one for converting dollars or euros into sterling; if the exchange rate is big, then you get a lot of dollars for your sterling. The value of c^2 happens to be very big indeed (about a hundred thousand trillion). If it were money, then one British pound would buy you a hundred thousand trillion dollars.

Einstein's equation tells us that every unit of mass gets you a hundred thousand trillion units of energy. You might now understand the desire in the early 20th century to 'split the atom.'

That is, to turn the mass of a heavy substance (like uranium or plutonium) into energy. Given the exchange rate, a nuclear reactor with just a small amount of uranium can power an entire country.

Use the Force

So, what about a physical law that might have an equivalent in consciousness? An obvious starting point is to take a law that describes how two things interact with each other in the physical world and see if we can write something equivalent in an equation for the way the consciousnesses of two people interact. Gravity governs the structure of the universe and how objects – planets, stars, and galaxies – interact with each other, so that seems like a good place to start.

Gravity

Gravity is everywhere; its universal presence is called the gravitational field. If we continue with the idea that matter is how consciousness appears, then we could try to think of a field of consciousness in a similar way to the gravitational field. We could consider that there's a field of consciousness that's also everywhere. In fact, this idea is actually consistent with nonduality: a single, infinite, unified consciousness.

Even though the gravitational field is universal – it's everywhere – things also have their own gravity. We usually talk about the gravity of the Earth because that's the only gravity we ever notice, but you and I have gravity; insects have gravity, apples and oranges have gravity. You don't notice your own gravity because it isn't strong enough to make apples zoom out of the fruit bowl toward you when you walk into the kitchen.

Your gravity is related to your mass. There's an equation in math that says so. The more there is of something, the more massive it is, then the more gravity it has. The Earth is much more massive than you, so it has a lot more gravity than you. It's why you fall back down again after you jump up, rather than the Earth coming up to meet you.

But gravity also gets weaker the further you move away from the Earth. The math equation for gravity says this too. It says that it weakens by the square of the distance you move away. If you go up really high, for example, almost into space, the Earth's gravity becomes so weak that you can float around weightlessly.

The equation can be written in English. It says that the gravity between two things – between the Earth and a person, say – is related to the mass of the Earth times the mass of the person, divided by the square of the distance between the Earth and the person.

In an equation, this is: $F = Gm_{Earth}m_{person}/d^2$. Here, F means the force of gravity, m is for the masses (with subscripts corresponding to the mass of the Earth and the mass of the person), d is for the distance between the person and the Earth, and G is the exchange rate (it's called the Universal Gravitational Constant).

The Consciousness Equation

Let's now imagine a field of consciousness, as with the gravitational field, but with each person and thing having their own field of consciousness too. So each person (and animal, bird, fish, insect, plant, rock, crystal, cloud, planet, star, and so on) has their own field of consciousness, just as they each have their own gravitational field.

And if we were to make an assumption that there's a direct comparison between gravity and consciousness, in that the law of gravity is an appearance of consciousness, then we might be able to say that the consciousness between two people will depend on the amount of each of their consciousnesses divided by the square of some measure of distance between them.

Now, physical distance isn't important. Consciousness is subjective so we need a subjective measure of distance, not an objective one. We could think of the *emotional distance* between two people – how connected they *feel* to each other.

And what about a subjective version of mass? Well, mass is a measure of the amount of something, so we might then think of an *amount of consciousness*. This could be expressed in different ways. We could think of it as an amount of intention, or an amount of belief or faith, or even an amount of intuition. These are all valid subjective ways of thinking of an amount of consciousness.

So we could say that the consciousness between two people, let's call them person A and person B, or Alice and Bob, would be related to the amount of Alice's consciousness times the amount of Bob's consciousness, divided by the square of the emotional distance between them. In an equation this would be:

$$S = \frac{C\, a_{Alice} a_{Bob}}{d^2}$$

S is for strength of interaction, C is the exchange rate (we'll explore this more in the next chapter), and the letter 'a' is for the amount of consciousness. I could have chosen any letter for the latter, but 'a' for amount made sense; however, we could use 'b' for the amount of belief, or 'i' for the amount of intuition or intention.

So, the strength of interaction between Alice and Bob (or any two people, animals, plants, objects, and so on) is related to the amount of their respective consciousnesses divided by the square of the emotional distance (or felt connection) between them.

What Does the Consciousness Equation Tell Us?

We now have two sentences, in English and math: one for the strength of gravity between two things (or people) and one for the strength of consciousness between two people (or things) – and they're essentially the same.

The first is a physical law of space-time about how two things interact, and the second is an equivalent 'law of consciousness' about how two consciousnesses interact. If it does turn out to be true that the physical world is how consciousness appears, then the two equations might work in a similar way. Here's how.

Think about what this consciousness equation tells us. The first thing to notice is the square of the emotional distance. This means that the further away Alice and Bob feel from each other emotionally, the weaker the interaction will be between their consciousnesses. This is common sense when you think about it: it's just like gravity – the further away you get from the Earth, the weaker you feel its gravity.

On the other hand, if Alice and Bob feel a strong connection with one another – that is, there's only a small emotional distance between them – then there will be a much stronger interaction between their consciousnesses.

So the equation tells us that the more connected two people feel, the more strongly their consciousnesses will interact. In effect, the equation seems to sensibly describe a real-world situation, which is often a good sign that an equation is on the right track.

The next thing to notice is that if either Alice or Bob, or both, have a large amount of consciousness, which could be a strong intention, belief, or intuition, then it also increases the interaction of their consciousnesses. So the greater our intention or belief (or faith), the more likely it is that our consciousness is felt by another person. By the same token, the greater our intuition, the more likely we are to sense another person's consciousness.

It's All About Emotional Connection

What's most important: emotional connection or amount of consciousness? They're both important, but emotional connection is the one that produces the biggest gains because it gets squared. It's the same with gravity – which is more affected by the distance between two things than by their masses.

The mass matters, of course, but the distance between them matters a bit more. And so the amount of consciousness a person brings – whether intention, belief, or intuition – matters, but the emotional connection makes more of a contribution.

So, how does this play out with people? Do you ever feel that you know when something's up in the life of a person to whom you feel strongly connected? Have you ever just *had a feeling*, say, that something bad had happened and it had? Yet you don't get the same strength of knowing with people you don't feel connected to?

Of course, we still get intuitions about things where emotional connection doesn't seem to be a factor, but this can be related to the amount of consciousness involved, which is likely to be the amount of our own intuition. Thus, being a highly intuitive person would help you intuit things even when emotional connection doesn't appear to be a factor.

It also suggests that saying a prayer or holding a compassionate intent (which we'll discuss in the next chapter) might have an effect on the person you're praying for, and that the strength of that effect will be related to how connected you feel to them. And if lots of people say the same prayer for the same person, so that the amount of consciousness is larger, then the strength of the impact on the person will also increase – even more so if they all feel a connection.

It also means that you needn't be concerned about a person having 'bad thoughts' about you. These won't affect you because if they're thinking of you in that way, there can't be much emotional connection in this instance. Emotional connection is about love, empathy, and compassion – a positive felt connection. Without that felt connection, the impact of a person's consciousness on yours will be little to nothing at all.

Unless, of course, you *believe* that their thoughts will affect you, which initiates the nocebo effect I mentioned in Chapter 1. Here, it's not a person's thoughts about you that are having a negative effect, but your *belief* that they are.

Emotional Entanglement

There's one other thing I wish to draw your attention to. There's no letter in the consciousness equation for physical distance.

This is because, as far as the interaction between two people's consciousnesses is concerned, the equation predicts that the physical distance between them is irrelevant.

It shouldn't matter at all whether Alice and Bob are standing right beside each other or are 1,000 miles apart. The strength of consciousness between them should be the same; for example, the impact of a prayer or the strength of an intuition should be the same regardless of the physical distance between them.

We might think of an 'emotional entanglement' or an 'entanglement in consciousness,' irrespective of physical distance, that mirrors the physical phenomenon of 'quantum entanglement,' which is where two particles once connected and then separated remain connected, regardless of the physical distance between them.

The same might be said, then, of two people who remain emotionally connected, even if one of them travels several thousand miles away. They still feel the same. In this way, if the physical world is indeed an appearance of consciousness, like gravity, the phenomenon of entanglement might also be an appearance of consciousness.

I sometimes picture this in my mind as a vast 3D web that connects all people and all things. In this web, the thickness of any one strand represents the emotional connection between people, so you'd barely see any strands connecting you with most people and things, but they're there all the same, like superfine wisps.

However, there are thick strands connecting you with the people with whom you do feel a bond, whether they're family, friends, or loved ones, and perhaps even with people you've not yet met but who are likely to play an important role in your life.

I've made this latter point because research suggests that physical entanglement between subatomic particles seems to transcend time. If the parallels I've suggested so far are on the right track, then the same might be true of connections with people we've not yet physically met.

Understanding the 'Field of Consciousness'

Let me expand on the concept of a field of consciousness before we move on to the next chapter. As I explained earlier in this chapter, everything has a field of consciousness, just as everything has a gravitational field. And, just as gravitational fields concentrate where there are greater amounts of matter, like plants and stars, so fields of consciousness concentrate in places where there are greater amounts of consciousness.

I'd now like to add to the suggestion I made earlier regarding *amounts* of consciousness. We might think of these amounts not only in terms of intention, belief (or faith), or intuition, but also self-awareness – that is, awareness of yourself as a conscious being.

If you were to visualize consciousness as light (which many people like to do), then everything and everyone in the landscape of the world around you would be glowing to some degree or other; some things (and people) would glow brightly and others would shine only faintly.

Before we go any further, in case you're having difficulty picturing a *field*, think of a fridge magnet. Its magnetic field is how far out you can feel its magnetism. It usually stretches a couple of centimeters; if you hold a paper clip close to it, you'll feel it pulled toward the magnet, but if you hold it a little further away, then the pull is much weaker.

Just like gravity, the strength of the magnetic field at any distance from the magnet is related to the square of the distance between the magnet and the paper clip. This 'inverse square law,' as it's known, is a law that a lot of natural phenomena seem to obey.

Your field of consciousness, then, is the distance out from you that it can be felt; but again, we're speaking of consciousness so it's a subjective measure of distance – it's about emotional distances or a sense of felt connection.

The Enlightenment Equation

The equation for the gravitational field is a lot like the equation for the force of gravity. If we were to write the equivalent for a field of consciousness, it would be equal to the amount of consciousness divided by the square of some distance in consciousness. So for Alice, it would be the amount of her consciousness divided by the square of some distance in consciousness, and we'd have an exchange rate as before:

$$C_f = \frac{C\,a_{Alice}}{d^2}$$

The only difference between this and the consciousness equation is that it doesn't include Bob's amount of consciousness, and that's because it's Alice's field of consciousness we're interested in.

I've chosen 'C_f' for 'field of consciousness' here. But what's the emotional distance this time? We can think of it in two ways.

It's actually the distance in consciousness – the felt connection – between Alice and any object of her attention. In the previous section, this object was Bob, but it can really be anything.

Suppose, then, that instead of using the distance in consciousness between Alice and another person, like Bob, we use the distance in consciousness between Alice and the infinite, unified, whole consciousness – or the universe, or even God, depending on how you think of it (or him or her).

The distance, now, is Alice's felt connection with the universe. It means that the more Alice feels connected to the universe, the smaller the distance in consciousness becomes between her and the universe, then the bigger and stronger her field of consciousness becomes. The greater her felt connection, the brighter she glows, if you were visualizing it as light.

Something very interesting happens when Alice feels herself to be so deeply connected that she's 'at one' with the universe, or in complete alignment as some would describe it. At that moment when her first-person experience is the feeling of being *at one*, the emotional distance effectively reduces to zero.

The equation tells us that, in that instant, Alice's field of consciousness becomes infinite. She becomes the universe in her felt experience. She might then describe herself as 'I Am.' This tallies with the experience of those people who have had near-death experiences, as we discussed earlier, who felt themselves to be infinite and at one with the universe. It also tallies with numerous spiritual writings, both ancient and modern.

Nonduality and idealism teachings tell us that this 'I Am' is our true nature, even if in everyday life it doesn't generally feel that way. Some call this kind of experience enlightenment – in the *light* of consciousness. We might call this new equation, then, the enlightenment equation.

Expanding the Field of Consciousness

In his book *The Power of Now* modern spiritual teacher Eckhart Tolle describes enlightenment as a state of 'felt one ness.' He also guides us in the importance of this when he writes that 'you find peace not by rearranging the circumstances of your life, but by realizing who you are at the deepest level.'[11]

An anonymous Native American saying declares, 'If we look at the path, we don't see the sky. We are Earth people on a spiritual journey to the stars. Our quest, our Earth walk, is to look within, to know who we are, to see that we are connected to all things, that there is no separation, only in the mind.'

There's no actual separation between things. Even Einstein's theory of relativity, which I touched on in the previous chapter, tells us that there's no absolute distance in space or time. We only have our experience, even if it seems consistent between us. The seeming separation between you and me, between you and the animals, birds, fish, insects, all of nature, is a perception, or some might call it an illusion.

There's no absolute separation between anyone or anything. There's only separation in a person's (felt or observed) experience. Kastrup wrote that we're dissociated alters (personalities) of the infinite consciousness, but dissociated only in our conscious experience, not at all in the truth of who or what we are.

The feeling of enlightenment is to feel *in the light of* the infinite consciousness, to feel at one with everything – God, the universe, or whichever description you prefer. The truly enlightened person's field of consciousness therefore is vast – not in physical size, of course, but in its magnitude.

It's been said that when an enlightened person arrives in a village, she or he will shift the consciousness of the whole village, and that people who come near will feel their field of consciousness even before any words are spoken. Some have dismissed such a thing as folklore, but it may well be representative of a truth.

How do we move toward this felt experience? The enlightened teachers who are written about in spiritual texts suggest that it's really quite simple. Love one another. Practice empathy. Show compassion. Be kind.

> *As we extend empathy and compassion outward to all people, animals, birds, insects, nature, life, we close the seeming gap between us.*

Emotional distance reduces. Love, empathy, compassion, and kindness therefore bring us together and cause us to feel connected with the universe as well as to the people, animals, and objects that we love, feel compassion for, or show kindness toward.

Aggression, hostility, and judgment, on the other hand, separate people and things, separate us from the universe in felt connection, and shrink a field of consciousness. Any way in which you can help to unite people, whether in your household, community, place of work, or further afield, reduces emotional distances and expands fields of consciousness. People who seek to divide others only shrink their own field.

If we come together as brothers and sisters on this planet and recognize each other as kin we collectively expand our human field of consciousness. In a sense, we 'ascend' to higher levels of consciousness.

But this isn't like attending a school or university where we graduate to higher levels by collecting knowledge. A person who has never attended school or read a book but who treats people with compassion can become enlightened in a heartbeat. Yet a person who has read a thousand spiritual books and has several university degrees but who treats people with unkindness or disrespect, as if they're superior, will have a very long wait.

If you truly want to feel enlightened, practice compassion. The goal of this shouldn't be enlightenment, however. Let *real* compassion be the goal. Only then will emotional distance be removed. Enlightenment is a side effect of it. Care. Be kind. Love one another, animals, and nature.

His Holiness the Dalai Lama sums it up in his book *Ethics for the New Millennium*: 'This, then, is my true religion. In this sense, there is no need for temple or church, for mosque or synagogue, no need for complicated philosophy, doctrine, or dogma. Our own heart, our own mind, is the temple. The doctrine is compassion.'[12]

CHAPTER 9

Telepathy, Distant Healing, and Prayer

In 1963, at Jefferson Medical College in Philadelphia, USA, identical twins sat in separate rooms 20 feet (6 meters) apart. One twin had been instructed to close their eyes at a set time to generate alpha brain waves – this is a well-known method of eliciting these waves. The Jefferson scientists wanted to know if the brain waves of the twin in the other room would also be in alpha in that instant.[1]

Out of 15 pairs of twins tested, two pairs were found to show a correlation in their brain waves. When one twin closed their eyes and their brain waves were recorded, the brain waves of their twin showed the same alpha brain wave pattern at precisely the same time.

The scientists also compared subjects who were unrelated and found there were no correlations at all. It wasn't being genetically identical that created the alpha wave synchronization, however.

Identical twins share much more than genetics – they tend to share a very strong emotional connection.

Researchers at the National Autonomous University of Mexico showed something similar to the twins study. Having recognized that emotional connection seemed to be the important factor, they tested EEG correlations between a psychotherapist and patients and discovered that the degree of correlations between them were in proportion to the degree of empathy between them.[2]

In a follow-up experiment published in the *International Journal of Neuroscience*, the researchers invited pairs of volunteers to sit side by side and try to feel one another's presence by generating a sense of empathy for each other. As they did so, their brain waves were measured.[3]

Then one volunteer in the pairing was moved to another room, where there was no possibility they could communicate with the other, while the brain waves were still being recorded. After a short while, that person had a light flashed in their eye. The EEG showed a specific pattern due to this 'visual stimulation,' yet at that instant the EEG of the person they'd previously sat with showed the same pattern.

Emotional Connection and Telepathic Ability

This phenomenon is called telepathy, or the less mystical-sounding 'correlations between the neural states of people who are separated by a distance.' Telepathy is often referred to as pseudoscience, in part because the assumption is that telepathic individuals sense thoughts as whole sentences and have long verbal conversations in their mind. That might be how it is in the movies, but real telepathy is much more subtle.

Although it's a taboo subject in science, there's quite a lot of evidence in support of telepathy, and emotional connection seems to matter quite a lot. An extremely impressive example of this was reported by Cambridge University professor Sir Rudolph Peters.[4] It involved a mother and her son, who had severe disabilities and with whom she shared an extremely strong emotional connection. Parents who care for, or have cared for, a child who is sick or has a disability know that the connection they feel with them is intensified by the many hours of dedicated care they give.

The mother had taken her son for an eye test because his sight was very poor, but he seemed to be able to read the letters on the Snellen eye chart much better than he should have. Intrigued, the optician asked the mother to leave the room, at which point the child's test results deteriorated considerably. Had the woman been giving her son some kind of hand signals to assist him? It seemed unlikely.

When Peters learned about this incident, he invited the mother and son to participate in an experiment. The pair sat in different labs that were around 5 miles (8 kilometers) apart and the mother was shown sequences of letters and numbers and the child had to guess what the letters and numbers were.

The boy's success rate was beyond astonishing – he guessed with an accuracy whose odds against chance were more than a billion to one. At the opticians he could apparently read the letters on the eye chart because the connection between him and his mother was so strong, he could *sense* what she could see.

Telepathy Studies

In an interview with *New Scientist* magazine, biologist and former Cambridge University don Rupert Sheldrake said that his studies showed that on the whole, women tend to be better at telepathy than men.[5] This tallies well with emotional connection: Women tend to be naturally more empathetic than men.[6]

It's believed that the gender difference evolved in the human species partially on account of women being primary caregivers and needing to develop an ability to read the state of an infant from nonverbal facial cues. As a result, over eons of time, we see today that women tend to rate a little higher in empathy than men. Of course, this is a generalization and shouldn't be taken as a truth about any one individual.

Empathy reduces emotional distances, so – as is consistent with the consciousness equation (*see page 184*), where a closer connection in this context equates to a higher likelihood of intuitive information received – we'd expect women to be better at telepathy than men. Therefore, emotional connection is the most important factor.

> *The higher a person is in empathy, the better we'd expect them to be at receiving telepathic sensations.*

Sheldrake also reported that children tend to be better than adults at telepathy and that people in traditional, non-Western societies seem to be better at it than people in Western societies, and especially better than well-educated people, who, he indicated, may have stronger skeptical beliefs. It may be that we do indeed have innate telepathic abilities but our over-reliance on modern means of communication drowns them out, in a similar way to how human magnetoreception has also become largely subconscious.

In his book *The Lost World of the Kalahari*, about the plight of the South African Bushmen, Laurens van der Post describes having been on a hunting expedition in the late 1950s with the Bushmen.[7] Van der Post asked one of the Bushmen how the people would react when they returned to the camp – which was about 50 miles (80 kilometers) from where the expedition had taken them – and learned that the hunt had been successful.

'They already know,' the man replied with utter sincerity.

'They know by wire. We Bushmen have a wire "here,"' he went on, tapping his chest in the area of his heart, 'that brings us news.' When the group finally returned to the camp, the people were indeed already celebrating the hunt's success.

Sheldrake has conducted a large amount of telepathy research. As an example, over several hundred tests, volunteers were asked to choose four people, either relatives or close friends, one of whom was randomly selected to phone the volunteer at an allotted time. When the phone rang, the volunteer had to guess which of the four was calling (this was in the days before caller ID).[8]

Chance would be that the volunteer would correctly guess about 25 percent of the time, but Sheldrake's studies had a guess rate of 42 percent. The statistical odds of this being anything other than a real phenomenon are astronomical (one hundred trillion trillion to one). And Sheldrake reported that the results were even stronger when the call came from someone with whom the volunteer had a very close bond.

This phenomenon even extends to the animals with whom we share an emotional connection. In his book *Dogs That Know When Their Owners Are Coming Home*, Sheldrake describes experiments where dogs were filmed becoming excited and running to the window at the exact moment their owner made the clear decision to leave their workplace.[9] In each case, he'd sent a text message to the person at a random time and asked them to make the clear decision, at that moment, to set off for home. Immediately, the CCTV cameras showed the dog moving to the window as if to greet their owner.

Spooky Action at a Distance

A University of Hawaii study used MRI scanners to study the seeming connections between people.[10] Eleven healers were invited to select someone with whom they felt a connection, and each person then lay inside an MRI scanner. At random intervals, and for two minutes each time, the healer sent healing intentions to the person from a distance away. The receiver didn't know when the healing was being sent, but there was activation in several brain regions at the precise times the healer sent their healing intention and not at any other times.

The healers used a variety of different healing methods, including reiki, qigong, Peruvian shamanic healing, Healing Touch, pule (a traditional form of prayer and chant usually performed by a Kahuna, a Hawaiian elder), vibrational or sound healing, plus three types that didn't fit into established known traditions.

Most healing practices are founded on a compassionate wish to help spare a person from suffering, so it likely doesn't matter that much who or what a healer believes in, or even which specific technique they use, so long as they feel compassion when they send healing and their intentions are honest and heartfelt.

A study conducted by a group of physicists attempted to investigate whether these connections, if real, could be explained by something like quantum entanglement between the brains of people separated by a distance.[11]

Entanglement is often referred to as 'spooky action at a distance,' a quip made by Einstein in a challenge to the accepted interpretation of quantum mechanics. It concerns the way subatomic particles that were once connected can remain connected (entangled), no matter how far apart they are – even if they're at opposite ends of the universe. Quantum mechanics predicted that a connection would exist regardless of the distance between them, which has now been experimentally proven correct.

Connecting Two Brains

As the brain is ultimately made of particles, the physicists hypothesized that some form of connection could show up between the brains of two people. Pairs of volunteers were invited to get to know each other and then sit together in meditation for 20 minutes. They were asked to try to *feel* one another's presence and to do so even if the physical distance between them changed.

The assumption was that this would facilitate some emotional connection and perhaps physical entanglement between the particles exchanged between their brains. In a control group, volunteers simply met with each other briefly but made no attempt to form an emotional connection. So felt connection was the difference between the two groups of volunteers.

Afterward, one of the pair was moved to an electromagnetically shielded room 48 feet (14.5 meters) away, and both volunteers had their brain state monitored by EEG. The shielded room was to rule out the possibility of connection by any physical means. Next, at random intervals, one of the volunteers was shown a series of light flashes for 2–5 seconds at a time, while the person they were trying to maintain a felt connection with stayed in the shielded room.

In the volunteers who had shared the meditative experience beforehand, there were clear correlations between their neural states in one out of four cases. At the instant of the light flash, the brain of the other person reacted. There were no correlations in the control group. The physicists wrote that the result, '… leaves no room for doubt about the existence of an unusual phenomenon, namely propagation of influence without local signals.' The term 'local signals' refers to any conventional means of information being sent.

Based on knowledge of the physicists' study and the seeming importance of emotional connection, Bastyr University and University of Washington scientists in the USA invited two people who had known each other as colleagues for two years to sit in meditative silence together for 10 minutes and also try to feel a connection between themselves.[12] They were to acknowledge that they were friends and colleagues and allow themselves to experience what that feels like by drawing their attention to it.

Then, one of the pair lay inside an MRI scanner while the other sat in a room located almost 33 feet (10 meters) away. At random times, the person in the room was shown a checkerboard pattern while the person in the scanner had their brain scanned.

Each time the person viewed the pattern, there was simultaneous activation in the visual cortex of their colleague in the MRI scanner (the visual cortex is the brain region that processes visual signals). In other words, one person saw something, yet the brain of the other person seemed to acknowledge it too. It was in some ways a shared experience.

When the volunteers swapped positions, however, the experiment didn't reveal a correlation. The authors suggested that any 'transmission' wasn't necessarily transitive; that is, flow in one direction doesn't necessarily imply flow in the other. Now, it's easy to be skeptical and simply conclude that if it didn't go both ways then the whole thing was just chance. But taking this position can miss something very important about the phenomenon.

The Transmission of Emotions

The result of the Bastyr University and University of Washington study is consistent with work on emotional connection in general, and with emotional contagion in particular. Emotional contagion is facilitated by the mirror neuron system (MNS) of the brain. As we discussed a little in Chapter 5, this is where a person can 'catch' the emotions of another person. It's related to empathy and, crucially, emotional contagion research shows that whether a person 'catches' an emotion from another depends on how each person feels about the other.

In other words, if Alice likes Bob, then Alice is likely to catch Bob's emotions because she has an empathetic sense for him; however, if Bob doesn't feel the same way about Alice – if he has no empathetic sense for her – then there's little chance that Bob will catch Alice's emotions. So, emotional contagion will flow from Bob to Alice but not necessarily from Alice to Bob. With any two people, emotional contagion quite often only goes one way and not the other. It's not necessarily transitive.

> *Generally speaking, emotional contagion*
> *(or transference) to you depends on your felt*
> *connection with the person you catch it from.*

Population studies involving the transmission of happiness and depression throughout the social networks of several thousand people show the same kind of effect. In one large study led by researchers at Harvard and Yale universities in the USA, happiness and even depression were shown to flow in one direction but not necessarily in the other, and the result was dependent on how one person felt about the other.[13]

The Bastyr University and University of Washington study was subsequently replicated using both EEG and MRI, and the same correlations were obtained. In one replication, 30 pairs of people who reported emotional connections with each other were examined using the same kind of setup. Five out of the 30 pairs showed significant correlations in neural activity.[14]

Despite their results occasionally being labeled pseudoscience, researchers in the field are convinced of their validity. They believe that further work shouldn't be concerned with whether or not the phenomenon is real, because the reality is pretty clear to them. Rather, it should focus on how it works, whether it exists in different populations of people with varying kinds of connections between them, and whether there are any clinical applications.

In other words, if a phenomenon shows up enough times, research should focus on what conditions are present when it does so, and even if there are particular types of people who have traits that are more conducive to it, or genes that make it more likely, or even if a person's mental health or life circumstances have a bearing on it.

And if emotional connection is important, then there should naturally be some people who are better at feeling emotional connection than others.

Love Connects

In an article titled 'The Return of Prayer' published in the journal *Alternative Therapies in Health and Medicine*, physician and author Larry Dossey writes that 'Love seems to function as a form of intercession – literally, a go-between – that unites the subject and the object being influenced.'[15] His investigations into prayer and distant healing showed that love could make quite a difference because it closed emotional gaps between subject and object.

In another paper called 'What's Love Got to Do With it?' Dossey shares examples of what the neurologist Berthold E. Schwarz referred to as telesomatic events.[16] These are where people who are separated by a distance seem to behave as a single person – such that one seems to sense when something has happened to the other by feeling it themselves. Schwarz had gathered over 300 examples, many from his patients.

Dossey noted that these telesomatic events tended to occur between people who shared loving and empathetic bonds, such as those between 'parents and children, siblings (particularly identical twins), spouses, and lovers.'[17] In one example, a mother had been writing a letter to her daughter when, all of a sudden, her right hand started to burn – so severely that she couldn't hold the pen. She received a phone call a short time later from the college that her daughter was attending to tell her that her daughter's right hand had been severely burned by acid. And it turned out that the accident had occurred at the same time that the mother's hand had begun to burn.

In another example, a woman suddenly doubled over in pain, clutching her chest. She said, 'Something has happened to Nell [her daughter]. She has been hurt.' The sheriff came by a few hours later and shared the news that Nell had been involved in a car accident and that a piece of the steering wheel had penetrated her chest.

Despite the seemingly mystical nature of these kinds of events, Dossey noted that 'they are quite common. Almost everyone seems either to have experienced them or to know someone who has.' We just tend not to speak of them for fear of what others will think of us – all the while unaware that those 'others' have also probably had similar experiences.

One morning, I experienced a recurring and rather imposing vision of a hole in some organic body substance. As the morning wore on, I realized that this repetitive, intrusive vision was a heart and that I was seeing a hole in it. And I say intrusive because the image kept spontaneously appearing in my mind's eye. To be honest, I panicked – I was scared that I was seeing a hole in my own heart. But I soon had an intuitive sense – which I know sounds woo-woo – that it wasn't my heart I was seeing.

I started to worry that it was someone in my family, so I spent much of the day offering silent prayers for various family members and phoning round to check that everyone was okay – inconspicuously, so as not to alarm anyone. Later that day, we received a phone call to let us know that my cousin's baby son had just been born, and that he had a small hole in his heart. The surgeons were able to repair it, though, and he made a full recovery.

Distant Healing Intention

The name given in research to therapies in which one person directs a mental healing intention toward another person is distant healing intention (DHI). It can have a religious or spiritual element, in which case it usually tends to be referred to as prayer.

Distant healing and prayer have been extensively researched in science. In these studies, people typically send healing intentions to other people, plants, or even biological organisms. There's some skepticism in the mainstream, because while many studies show a clear effect of distant healing or prayer, some show little or sometimes no effect at all. It's natural to be skeptical, then, and imagine that if the phenomenon doesn't show up all of the time then it's not real because it's not reproducible.

This attitude is captured well in the results of a Cochrane review into the efficacy of prayer.[18] It concluded that there was no convincing evidence for the efficacy of prayer. The authors wrote, 'These studies are equivocal and, although the results of individual studies suggest a positive effect of prayer, the majority don't, and the evidence does not support a recommendation either in favor or against the use of intercessory prayer.'

But the problem is, since our idea of prayer tends to be of petitioning a deity to intervene to help someone, it doesn't occur to many researchers to include any form of emotional connection in their study protocols. So we find that some prayer studies do involve emotional connection, where researchers have tended to be aware of its importance, and some don't. And on the whole, the results of the efficacy of prayer tend to be stronger when there is emotional connection and less so in its absence.

The Cochrane review considered a large number of studies but selected 10 for formal analysis – these were the ones that best met the statistical and study quality requirements. Out of these 10 studies, a total of 7,646 sick patients were prayed for, and three studies showed clear positive results. One of these three allowed for emotional connection – a double-blind randomized controlled trial conducted by Randolph Byrd, M.D., from the cardiology division at the University of California at San Francisco and published in the *Southern Medical Journal* in 1988.[19]

Byrd's study involved 393 coronary care unit patients, 192 of whom were prayed for and 201 were in a control group for comparison. Prayers were offered by groups of Christians, selected from both Catholic and Protestant churches.

Each intercessor, as those offering the prayers are known, was asked to 'pray daily for a rapid recovery and for prevention of complications and death,' in addition to other areas of prayer they believed would be beneficial to the patient. They were given the first name, diagnosis, and the general condition of the patient they were to pray for. They were also given regular pertinent updates about their progress.

In the context of emotional connection, let's consider what the latter does. When you say a prayer for someone, the first time can feel a little detached – especially if you don't know the person or much about them – but if you're given regular updates about how they're getting on, you start to feel a connection with them.

They're no longer just a name or a number – they're a real person who is suffering and, hopefully, getting better. You start to form an emotional investment in their recovery.

In this study, the patients who were prayed for had an overall lower illness severity score (a measure of the severity of their condition) than patients who weren't prayed for. They also needed less ventilatory assistance, antibiotics, and diuretics than those who weren't prayed for. All in all, being prayed for seemed to help them.

When There's No Emotional Connection

Contrast this result with typical studies that show no evidence of the efficacy of prayer. I've chosen a large Duke University study as a representative example from the Cochrane review, whose protocol was similar to that of other studies which indicated that prayer was ineffective, as it's often cited in science as the definitive study that proved that prayer doesn't have any effect.[20]

In the study, 192 patients recovering from cardiac bypass surgery were prayed for and compared with a similar number of patients who weren't being prayed for. Prayers were given in two tiers, or phases, by prayer groups representing Christian, Muslim, Jewish, and Buddhist traditions.

For the first phase, intercessors were given each patient's name, age, and illness. For the second phase, additional intercessors were given no names or details but instead were asked to 'pray for the prayers of the primary tier congregations,' who were also offering prayers during this time. This study found no evidence that prayer was effective as there was no difference in cardiovascular outcomes between the patients who were prayed for and those who weren't.

A similar Harvard study found the same thing – no effect of prayer.[21] Coronary artery bypass graft patients had either been prayed for or not. Intercessors were given the first name and the first initial of the surname, plus an anonymous site code. Prayers were offered 'for a successful surgery with a quick, healthy recovery and no complications.'

Given that so much evidence exists for the importance of emotional connection, as we discussed earlier in this chapter, it seems to me that the Randolph Byrd study was more likely to work because it created a good opportunity for people praying to feel a connection with the people they were praying for.

The Missing Active Ingredient

I'd say that one of the reasons why the Duke and Harvard university studies didn't find any evidence for the efficacy of prayer is because there was no opportunity for emotional connection. This isn't intended as a criticism of these studies, nor of the Cochrane review; on the contrary, the Duke and Harvard study designs and execution were exemplary, as was the attention to detail and statistical analysis of the Cochrane review. These studies did exactly what they set out to do and were carried out to exacting standards.

I'm merely pointing out that the active ingredient missing in some studies that suggest distant healing or prayer don't work is emotional connection, and that it tends to be present in many of the successful studies. There are some exceptions, of course, but generally speaking, successful prayer studies tend to involve emotional connection, while unsuccessful ones don't. What should we ultimately conclude from this?

> **Prayer does work, but it tends to work better when the person praying is able to form some emotional connection with the person for whom they're praying.**

'Where does this leave God if emotional connection matters so much?' a Christian friend asked me recently. My response was along the lines of 'perhaps compassion, which fosters emotional connection, is God's language, so maybe it represents God working *through* you in your prayers.'

It may have been that a lot of researchers didn't realize at the time they designed their studies that emotional connection mattered, so they didn't include it in their method. And researchers skeptical of the phenomenon, who also sometimes conduct the studies, wouldn't naturally consider emotional connection to be important, given a starting materialist mindset that consciousness, if it exists at all, resides within the skull.

A distant intention is what researchers seek to measure, so the experiment is narrowed down to that active ingredient alone. This is of course the right thing to do, but only if you don't know that emotional connection is an active ingredient too – in fact, perhaps the most important one in the phenomenon you're trying to measure.

Also, when it comes to prayer, consider what that is to most people. The Cochrane review defined it as the 'solemn request or thanksgiving to God or object of worship.' In other words, as I said earlier, we petition God or another deity on behalf of someone who is in need. There's no assumption that some form of emotional connection is even necessary. All you need, technically, is the person's name or image so God knows who to help. Given this, why would prayer researchers give anything other than the person's name to those doing the praying?

It's when all else seems lost that many people, even those who have always rejected religion or spirituality, turn to prayer. And for those skeptical of prayer, praying for the surgeon or carers can feel more acceptable. A friend's father was seriously ill a few years ago and had to undergo an emergency operation. The family has a very strong faith and let the surgeon know that they would be praying for the father. The surgeon said, 'Why don't you pray for me, that I perform the best operation I can?'

Motivation to Heal

Most of us know from experience that motivation and some practice can help us improve at almost anything, whether it's a physical thing like a sport or a musical instrument or something cognitive like mathematics or crossword puzzles. Some research has shown that the same is true when people say prayers for others or send healing mentally. Motivation and training improve the results.

In his book *Real Magic*, Dean Radin, Chief Scientist at the Institute of Noetic Sciences, USA, pointed out that volunteers typically recruited for distant healing intention and prayer experiments aren't trained in how to focus.[22]

As we discussed earlier, we know from meditation research that focus on the breath alters the structure of the prefrontal cortex, making focusing easier, just as strength training of an arm muscle alters it and makes lifting objects easier. Anyone knows from experience that practice in focusing on something makes it easier to focus. This is, in part, due to practice-induced physical changes in the brain.

In prayer and distant healing intention studies, the volunteers are also not especially motivated. They're generally simply curious and are usually recruited via adverts and the promise of payment. Lastly, in studies, because of the way they're recruited, volunteers generally don't tend to share an emotional connection with any of the other volunteers. In fact, they usually don't know anyone else participating at all.

Think of it this way: if one of your loved ones was sick and you were praying for them, you'd be highly motivated and focused with your prayers, much more so than if you were part of an experiment that asked you to send healing mentally to a random person, and especially if you only knew the person's first name and the first initial of their surname.

> **The more motivated a person is, the more of their consciousness they focus on the healing.**

In the consciousness equation that I shared in the previous chapter, motivation to heal would affect the amount of consciousness focused on a person's healing, so it does matter – not as much as emotional connection, but it matters all the same.

Practice Helps

A double-blind study was set up that would ensure motivation to heal, training, and emotional connection – and the results were compelling.[23] The study involved 36 'bonded pairs.' These are people who share an emotional connection, in this case, long-term couples, mother-and-child pairs, and lifelong friends. In 22 pairs, one of the receivers was a cancer patient, for whom motivation was a given.

For the experiment, both individuals were asked to hold a feeling of being connected with their partner, what the researchers called compassionate intent. To aid the feeling, they were invited to hold a personal item belonging to the other in their hand, such as a ring, watch, or other small item.

The person receiving the intentions also learned that their partner would be able to see their live image on a screen. This also helped the volunteers establish and maintain a felt connection with each other. The autonomic nervous system (ANS) of the receiver was monitored throughout the experimental times.

Each day, the receiver relaxed for 30 minutes in an electromagnetically shielded room some distance away while compassionate intent was sent by their partner in random 10-second intervals at times unknown to the receiver. To test the effect of training, 12 of the senders had been asked to practice this daily for three months leading up to the experiment. This was called the trained group.

The results showed a very strong correlation between the ANS of the sender and receiver. Typically, the sender's ANS activity increased at the time they sent intention (it increased as a result of the mental effort, which is quite typical), and the receiver's ANS activity increased about a half second later. In other words, the nervous system of the receiver correlated with the feelings of the sender.

And, as predicted by the researchers, the effect was stronger in the couples where the sender had received prior training in sending the intention. It seemed that practice made people better at sending healing; either that or practice enhanced the ability to feel a connection. Or it may have been both.

Ultimately, the study showed that emotional connection matters and so does motivation to heal. Some training helps too. It makes sense that practice at sending healing intention will make a person better at doing so. This is most people's experience, so why should practice not be of importance in scientific experiments that involve feeling an emotional connection and wishing wellness in our prayers for someone?

Can Consciousness Influence Physical Things?

So far, I've talked about telepathy and of people sending healing intentions or prayers to other people, but if we continue to suppose that everything is part of a universal field of consciousness and everything *has* a field of consciousness, then a conscious intention should impact on anything, even if the effects are small.

Consequently, a lot of research has looked into whether conscious intention can impact physical systems instead of people or biological systems (such as plants or organisms). To be clear, it's easy to leap to the conclusion that if consciousness *can* somehow impact physical things, then we should all be able to levitate objects (and ourselves) with our mind, will a pencil to move across a table, and even bend a metal bar with the power of thought.

This is a common skeptical objection to the notion that consciousness can impact reality. The husband of a friend who had attended some of my lectures once alluded to this, saying: 'Since these things clearly don't happen, consciousness is obviously just a brain state and it can't affect anything outside the skull.' However, that's not what the scientific data shows. There *is* a subtle and undeniable influence of consciousness detectable even in inanimate physical things. The effect is small, but it's real all the same.

The Consciousness Constant

At this point, I'd like to return your attention to the 'exchange rate' term C in the consciousness and enlightenment equations (*see pages 184 and 190*); I've deliberately not said anything more about this until now. In mathematics and physics, these exchange rates are known as known as 'constants.'

The Universal Gravitational Constant, G, essentially reduces the number value of the force of gravity. G has a value of about a ten billionth. If it were 1 instead of a ten billionth, gravity would be so strong that we'd be squashed as flat as a pancake. G's number value reflects the fact that we tend to live without being squashed. You can think of it as a reducing (or damping) constant because its value reduces, or dampens, the force of gravity.

In the same way, I hypothesize that the constant C in the consciousness equation (we might call it the consciousness constant) does something similar to the force of consciousness for humans. It greatly reduces (dampens) the force of consciousness, so we don't typically levitate objects, will pencils to move across tables, or bend metal bars with our mind. If I were to guess, the value probably relates to the relative amount that the human species is in general 'dissociated' (to borrow Bernardo Kastrup's word) from the single whole of consciousness.

It's not that consciousness can't do amazing things – I suspect there's the odd person here or there who does seemingly exert stronger mental effects on objects – but for humans in general, the seeming power of consciousness to impact physical and biological matter is reduced so much by the constant C that the effects we see are generally small and subtle, but real all the same.

Consciousness-Matter Interaction

Typically, scientific studies that probe the impact of consciousness on physical matter use what are called RNGs (random number generators) – physical systems (computers) that generate bits of random data, typically at the rate of about 200 bits per second. The idea is that given the rate and volume of numbers, if consciousness could interact with matter then we might see statistically significant patterns of non-randomness at times when a conscious intention is focused. And this is exactly what happens.

The effect is especially pronounced when there's some form of emotional connection. Of course, it's hard to feel emotionally connected to a computer or some other metal device in the way we've understood it so far. But we can still feel connected. In the consciousness equation, I refer to it as 'emotional connection' only because I'm speaking about people. I also call it 'felt connection,' and say that it can be with any object of attention; people and the universe are just relevant examples.

Scientists sometimes call this kind of connection a sense of resonance, or a feeling of being at one with the thing, or feeling in alignment with it, especially in studies that examine an effect of consciousness.

Resonance

In his book *Real Magic*, Dean Radin discusses some of the research that was done into mind–matter interactions (with RNGs) at the University of Edinburgh in Scotland in the 1970s and 80s.[24] He says that the volunteers were asked which kind of strategies worked best for them and that the most successful strategy reported was a feeling of resonance, a feeling of being at one, with the RNG.

> *When a sense of connection exists, whether with a person or an object, some of the seeming separation in consciousness between them begins to dissolve.*

Ultimately then, it doesn't really matter whether the connection we feel is with a person, a spiritual deity, a device, a tree, or even a crystal. What matters is a sense of felt connection.

The Edinburgh University researchers also found that some of the volunteers reported success with other strategies, including asking entities (such as angels and guides) for help, using emotion to give the intention more power, focused concentration, relaxation, visual imagery, even speaking with the device as if it were a sentient being. But resonance, a sense of connection, was the most successful strategy.

Studies at Princeton University, in a division known as PEAR (Princeton Engineering Anomalies Research), which ran from the 1970s until 2007, found the same thing: a sense of 'resonance, immersion, with a loss of awareness of the self,' where we feel a sense of one ness with a person, deity, or object, was key.[25]

Absorption

Robert Jahn, former Dean of Engineering at Princeton University and then Director of the PEAR laboratory, wrote that the volunteer who was the most successful at impacting the RNGs reported that they 'simply fell in love with the machine.'[26] This can also be called absorption. Absorption is associated with a loss of awareness of time and space – being totally engrossed or immersed in, or connected with, what we're doing.

Research by psychologist Lonnie Nelson at the University of Arizona, USA, explored the idea further and discovered correlations between psi activity (a general term for paranormal or psychic phenomena) and absorption.[27] He found that the degree of absorption was correlated with the size of the effect. The more absorption there was – that is, the stronger the felt connection – the greater the degree of mind–matter interaction.

The study also compared results at two distances and found the effects were independent of distance and only dependent on the degree of absorption, which we might expect if the consciousness equation is on the right track. As I pointed out in Chapter 8, the consciousness equation doesn't have any variables (letters) for physical distance, so physical distance shouldn't make any difference.

More Than Chance

A study in Toronto, Canada, led by neurologist Morris Freedman, who had some healthy skepticism regarding psi, attempted to replicate some of the PEAR research.[28] He and his team chose subjects with frontal lobe brain damage. As Freedman pointed out, at the time there was well-established research literature showing that self-awareness is mediated by the frontal lobes, and that the presence of lesions there reduces it. Thus, these patients would feel a greater sense of absorption naturally.

Of the six subjects with brain damage, four had lesions in both frontal lobes; one had lesions on the right frontal lobe, and the other had lesions on the left frontal lobe. They were compared against six subjects without brain lesions.

Each subject was given an instruction: 'There are some people who believe that if we concentrate on something hard enough, we can affect how things happen. Now we don't know if this is true, but we have undertaken to test this out. We would like to see if there is a possibility that people can influence something just by concentrating on it.'

Then, as the subjects sat in front of a computer monitor, an arrow on the screen was moved according to a random number sequence that was generated at a rate of 200 bits per second, and the subjects were asked to try to will it to go either left or right.

The subjects did 10 blocks of 100 trials, which lasted around 15 minutes, and this was compared against 1,000 control trials with no one in the room. A significant effect was seen in the patient who had damage to the left frontal lobe when they attempted to move the arrow to the right. The result remained significant through rigorous statistical controls.

In a replication, again designed with tight statistical controls, the researchers specifically set out to test whether or not the patient with left frontal lobe lesions could mentally shift the arrow to the right. Again, the result was confirmed – this patient *was* able to mentally shift the arrow to the right. The researchers recommended that future work on studying the effects of consciousness on physical systems might consider involving patients with frontal lobe lesions.

The initial data was met with caution in the scientific community, and rightly so, as statistical aberrations can and do occur. But the researchers reported that 'the replication of the findings in the left frontal patient in a second well-designed study suggests that the effect in this subject may be more than chance occurrence.' This was a significant statement.

CHAPTER 10

The Right Conditions

On July 4, 2012, scientists at CERN (a research organization that operates the world's largest particle physics laboratory) announced the discovery of the Higgs boson, first predicted by Peter Higgs, Emeritus Professor of Theoretical Physics at the University of Edinburgh, Scotland.[1] Popularly known as the 'God particle,' the Higgs boson gives elementary particles their mass and its discovery confirmed a key prediction of the Standard Model of particle physics.

The confirmation of the Higgs boson after a 45-year search was met with cheer in the scientific community around the world, and Peter Higgs was awarded the Nobel Prize in Physics the following year. Proof that this really was the particle depended on statistics, but as the data exceeded the 'five sigma' threshold on the scale scientists use to describe the certainty of a discovery (which is five standard deviations from the mean and represents odds against chance of 1 in 3.5 million), the Higgs boson's existence was accepted as a scientific fact.

Yet, despite frequently being labeled pseudoscience, much of the data in support of psi (telepathy, precognition, RNGs, and other topics in the general field of parapsychology) exceeds the *six sigma* threshold (six standard deviations from the mean).[2] This represents odds of the phenomena being chance as greater than a billion to one – significantly in excess of the statistical evidence for the Higgs boson.

Unfounded Skepticism

While she was President of the American Statistical Association and addressing its annual conference of around 6,000 statisticians in 2016, Jessica Utts said: 'The data in support of precognition and possibly other related phenomena are quite strong statistically, and would be widely accepted if they pertained to something more mundane. Yet, most scientists reject the possible reality of these abilities without ever looking at the data.'[3]

Utts went on to describe some of the work she'd done in the psi field, including a year spent on a classified project for the US government during the Cold War. She'd written a report for the US Congress on this work and declared to the conference delegates that she stood by it to that day.

> *Ironically, dismissing something on the basis of a belief and without examining the data is itself pseudoscience, not the research that's being dismissed as pseudoscience.*

During my academic studies it was always drilled into me that we must examine the data and never say something simply because we've heard someone else say it or because we've read someone's opinion of it on a social media post. When the subject of telepathy, prayer, distant healing, presentiment, ESP, and other areas come up at social gatherings, I voice my positive opinion of it and that's usually well received, but on occasion I've met skepticism.

I also frequently hear (and read) statements like 'the complete nonsense that is parapsychology' or 'there's absolutely no evidence for psi.' Such views are often expressed by people who are well intentioned, but have nevertheless neither read any papers published in the field nor personally examined a single statistical analysis.

This bias has its roots in our ingrained materialist conviction that consciousness is an illusion, or at least locked in the skull and produced in some way (even if we don't understand it yet) by the brain. So it simply *must be* that the data is flawed in some way, or that the researchers are charlatans or at the very least misguided.

I honestly don't feel that this is very respectful. Scientists in these fields dedicate their lives and careers to studying and attempting to understand some of these mysteries of life, often showing tremendous courage in the face of skepticism, criticism, and sometimes ridicule. Whether their research turns out to be right or wrong, at least they're trying, and for that I feel we should grant them respect and not make sweeping dismissals of their work without having *read* any of it.

I do understand the skepticism, though, because I also occasionally hear people say things like 'If holding a positive intention for someone is all we need to do, we shouldn't also need drugs,' or

'Why is it that sick people die even when they've others thinking positive thoughts about them and praying for them?'

However, such sentiments are based on our assumption that parapsychology researchers are saying we can all levitate objects with our mind, will pencils to roll across tables, and just think a positive thought and all of our loved ones will be instantly healed. I wish it were that easy. But that's not what they're saying. They're telling us about a measurable effect of consciousness irrespective of physical distance – that we can sense things and that if we hold a compassionate intent for someone, we *can* sometimes help them.

A Fear of Endorsing PSI

I've made enquiries into the reasons behind skepticism of parapsychology research, and the responses have shone an interesting light on it. In addition to the above, they point toward the following: a) a fear that endorsing anything in the parapsychology field lends credence to the argument for the existence of a God who controls our lives; b) a fear of feeding into a magical, unscientific belief system and in so doing shattering some of the credibility of science; and c) a belief that consciousness is produced by the brain and so it's impossible for it to affect someone far away.

I do understand this reasoning. After all, science has shaped our world for the better in many ways. We have modern medicine and computers. We have an understanding of virus transmissions that helped us act quickly enough to reduce significantly the death toll from SARS-CoV-2 (coronavirus).

Some fear that science will suffer a loss of credibility if 'hippy' beliefs are given weight, and as a result, life-saving advice may not be taken as seriously. But at the same time, we shouldn't dismiss an area of research simply because we don't believe the phenomena it investigates is possible, or because we think some people might try to harness its findings in an unethical or less than healthy way. One of the pillars of science is to investigate and understand phenomena, not to dismiss it without looking at it.

PSI Research

As far as researchers in the field are concerned, parapsychological (psi) phenomena are real. They're no longer interested in trying to convince others, though – they're happy to let us fight about it and just get on with their own work. Today, researchers are more interested in what makes one person better at psi than someone else, and whether there are certain conditions and types of environments or circumstances in which the phenomena seems to be stronger.

One area where such research has moved on is presentiment – that is, gut feelings, intuition, a sense of the future. As this is quite subjective, scientists typically monitor a subject's nervous system to see if it responds *before* an event in a way that's not simply a chance anticipation.

For example, in numerous trials, volunteers sat facing a computer that made random selections of images from a database. The images were emotionally neutral, stimulating, or calm. Repeatedly, the human nervous system reacted to the nature of the image *before* the computer had even made a random selection, with a presentiment window, as it's called, of 3–5 seconds on average.

This means that under those conditions, the human nervous system had a sense of what was coming next, as if it had a window looking onto it, around 3–5 seconds before it actually happened. These studies show that animals display presentiment too, including dogs, cats, and even earthworms.

You might wonder if we just *anticipate* what might come next. If that was the case then the guess rate would be chance, but even after thousands of trials, the guess rate far exceeds chance. As with other psi research, the data is compelling. In discussing this and other general psi research, Dick Bierman, a Dutch psychologist with a background in molecular physics, wrote, 'We're satisfied that people can sense the future before it happens. We would now like to move on and see what kind of person is particularly good at it.'[4]

What Kind of People Are Adept at PSI?

The ability to sense danger before it happens would have been an advantage to our African savanna-dwelling ancestors. Individuals with an intuition that something dangerous lay ahead might walk the other way; sometimes that would save their lives and they'd be able to pass their genes on to the next generation, including the genes that lent them that ability to sense danger.

Think of a gene as having a color. Over time, genes undergo small mutations, so here, a gene can develop different shades, or variants, of the color. If it's a pink gene, say, then over time mutations might produce 50 shades, or variants, of pink, from baby pink all the way to deep pink, which is almost red.

Let's say it's a gene for kindness that influences how likely a person is to show kindness to someone who is suffering. Some people will have a gene that ensures they'll move pretty quickly to help the person, but others will have a gene variant that makes them less likely to help. This work has actually been done with kindness, where the likelihood of helping a person in need is correlated with a variant of the oxytocin (kindness hormone) receptor gene.

In terms of psi, if there *are* genes related to psi ability, then different variants of the gene would be distributed among us, just as the variants of the oxytocin receptor gene are. Some people will be naturally adept at things like sensing the future, telepathy, and sending distant healing, and some will not. And nature and nurture are also at play. As with all genes, some people with natural psi ability may have had it developed while others may have had it quashed; and some with little ability may have had it encouraged or negated.

> *In some psi experiments, there are a small number of people who score repeatedly higher than everyone else.*

Therefore, they may well have a positive gene variant for it but their individual ability sometimes gets lost in the statistics, which tend to average the scores of all participants. For example, if a psi experiment involved 100 people and one person scored 80 percent while 99 people scored about 50 percent, the average score would be 50.3 percent. This is essentially rounded down to 50 percent and the result is deemed 'chance.' That one person's score of 80 is either averaged into the whole or is dismissed altogether and considered an error or 'outlier.'

Mistaken Conclusions

This isn't always the right way to go. What if there was something unique about the person who scored 80 percent? What if one in 100 people shared some trait that gave them a different kind of ability?

Imagine if we didn't know how fast humans could run but we wanted to know. If we took a sample of 1,000 people and timed them sprinting 100 meters, we might find that the average time would be around 20 seconds, with more than half of all the runners within a few seconds either side of this. We'd obtain a bell-shaped curve centered on a mean of 20 seconds.

We might then conclude that humans can run 100 meters in around 20 seconds. Yet Usain Bolt ran it in 9.58 seconds. We don't think of this situation as being the same, though, because it's something we're familiar with. Obviously, some humans can run 100 meters in under 10 seconds because we've witnessed it on live TV! But in psi and other statistical studies, Bolt's result would be averaged out into the mean of all 1,000 people and would be forgotten about.

We might not believe any of the anecdotal stories about runners clocking 9.6 seconds or less and might even dismiss published results of under 10 seconds as down to faulty timing or even fraudulent behavior by charlatans. After all, the number of people who say they can run 100 meters in under 10 seconds is a very small number compared with the general population.

We'd conclude that no human could run this distance in under 10 seconds; it's a preposterous idea. But this is what actually happens in psi (and other) experiments. In many other fields of science, we can (and do) easily miss phenomena when it appears to be far from the norm.

Potential Blocks to PSI Ability

It seems to me that some people are naturally more adept at psi – just as some people are naturally better runners and some people are naturally kinder – and we should invest time and effort into learning who they are and why that is, and which conditions are most conducive to psi. Given what we've explored so far, overly clinical conditions devoid of any emotional connection certainly don't seem to be conducive, so we could start with 'warmer' conditions that foster emotional connection.

In addition, I'm not sure that it's so easy just to switch on psi in the same way we turn on our ability to get up from a chair or speak a sentence. Most people who have had personal psi experiences will attest to the fact that they're quite spontaneous.

Writers, artists, musicians, and other creative people know that it can be difficult to sit down on cue and produce their best work. Often, it arrives at unexpected moments – when you're laughing with friends, listening to music, driving a car, sitting on a bus or a plane, walking in the park, watching TV, even while having a glass (or two) of wine. But for the most part, timing can be seemingly random. So, we need to design psi experiments that account for the spontaneous nature of the phenomena.

Incidentally, there's now evidence that artistic and creative people score better in psi experiments than the average person, so this might suggest there's some genetic effect.[5] Perhaps having a creative mind is an aid to psi. It might be, therefore, that an analytical mind could be a hindrance.

Given that scientific training is typically analytical, it might even be that scientists, while exceptionally talented in some arenas, represent a segment of the population who are particularly poor at psi. (I'm generalizing that people drawn to science are typically more analytically minded, although this isn't strictly the case.) Here, then, a general level of skepticism is therefore to be expected – based not just on ignorance of the data but also on real-world experience.

It's also likely that trained skepticism might block natural psi abilities. A fear of being ridiculed by their peers might account for the position that some scientists have on the matter. It takes enormous courage to declare an open-minded attitude toward something that so many view as pseudoscience. We're only human, after all.

If You Believe

So-called sheep–goat experiments compare the extrasensory perception (ESP) ability of people who believe in ESP against those who don't.[6] Overwhelmingly, sheep (believers) perform much better in these studies than goats (skeptics).

A meta-analysis of such experiments containing over half a million ESP guesses by 4,500 people gave odds against chance of more than one trillion to one. Believers in these kinds of studies really do score better than skeptics. As far as these analyses go, ESP ability is correlated with belief in ESP ability. It's like the placebo effect playing out with ESP.

With knowledge of this research in mind, I once conducted an experiment in a series of workshops in which audience members had to guess the color – either red or black – of 20 playing cards. I started out by enthusiastically sharing some of the science on ESP – a few experimental results, how I believe it works – and then asked the participants to write a few paragraphs as if they were explaining to a skeptic why ESP is real. My intention was to instill a belief in ESP, because if belief affects ability then we'd be more likely to see an ESP effect in the workshop.

In half a dozen workshops involving a few hundred people, the audience members correctly guessed the color of the cards about 56 percent of the time. The experiment was crude and I didn't have a comparison group – I'd never intended to publish it, as it was more about demonstrating the phenomenon to participants – but chance would have given 50 percent. It was a fun exercise, really, but I mention it here in the context of pointing out that a positive belief in psi seems to *enhance* psi ability.

How Experimenters Affect Experimentees

Given that we're studying consciousness, and how our fields of consciousness can mix and impact on each other and on physical systems, it seems to me that even the beliefs of the researchers who carry out experiments matter too. Their beliefs should influence their results in a few ways.

First, and most obviously, the attitudes, beliefs, and even subtle body language of experimenters affect the state of volunteers in a study and can influence what they expect. This is partly why pharmaceutical drugs trials are done double-blind – where not even the doctor or nurse knows who receives a drug or a placebo. And second, the state of consciousness (whether sheep or goat, believer or skeptic) of the experimenters might impact on the consciousness of the volunteers, or even on a physical system being used – enough to tilt the experiment in the direction of what the experimenters expect.

An interesting study, published in the *British Journal of Psychology*, involved a collaboration between a psi researcher and a skeptic of psi.[7] The aim was to attempt to influence mentally the autonomic nervous system of a person at a distant location. The psi researcher succeeded in his attempt, but the skeptic failed, although they had followed the exact same protocol.

Naturally, in science, we'd conclude that psi doesn't exist because the skeptic showed that the result wasn't replicated. So the believer must have made some kind of error. But what if it was the other way round, and the skeptic had made the error? Or, given that we're measuring the effects (if any) of consciousness, what if the skeptic's state of consciousness (their belief that it's all nonsense) influenced a null result?

This is a valid interpretation of the research to which we must be open. The consciousness of the person or people doing the research can't be separated from the experiment itself.

In physics, the concept that an experimental result can be tracked back to the consciousness of the experimenter is known as a von Neumann chain (or von Neumann-Wigner interpretation). It relates to observations of quantum mechanical systems in which the consciousness of an observer is thought to 'collapse the wave function' and determine an outcome being measured.

In psi studies, the consciousness of the experimenter is part of the experiment.

Ignoring it would be a bit like doing a sensitive experiment to measure the heat produced by an object and not taking into account the heat from the hands of the person handling it. Therefore, we have to assume that the consciousness of the experimenter – their belief in psi – can influence whether the result is positive or negative. So, whether or not they believe in psi could genuinely influence the result. There is mounting evidence to suggest that this is indeed the case.

In the previously described experiment, the psi researcher believed in psi, so their belief might have influenced the likelihood of a positive result, enough that the observed result was statistically significant. On the other hand, the skeptic didn't believe in psi and so this could have influenced a null result. As well as being a test of the reality of psi, the study may also have been a test of what each research group collectively *believed*.

Accounting for Consciousness

Another study used a more technically sophisticated physics setup and found a similar effect. It was conducted by scientists at the PEAR laboratory at Princeton University, who had previous experience of psi research and believed in psi.

Publishing in the journal *Cellular and Molecular Biology*, the PEAR researchers wrote: 'Another failed attempt at inter-laboratory replication involved a double-slit photon detector as a target. In this instance, the initial experiment was conducted by an optical physicist with a somewhat skeptical view of such anomalous phenomena, and produced only chance results. When his device was installed at the PEAR laboratory, however, significant extra-chance results were obtained following the same operational protocol.'[8]

Although they had used exactly the same equipment and experimental protocol, the researchers who believed in psi successfully measured an effect while the skeptical physicist didn't.

This 'non-replicability suggests false' approach is clearly correct in fields of science that don't investigate consciousness, but *we are* investigating consciousness, so our experiments and analyses must account for the state of consciousness of the people involved with the experiments. Perhaps, going forward, experimenters should declare themselves believers or skeptics, sheep or goats, and publish this alongside their research. That would give scientists an additional, and potentially helpful, stream of data.

Measuring What's Appropriate

Before we move on to the next chapter, I believe it's worth saying a few words about the strength of psi and why *what* we choose to measure in distant healing and prayer studies can influence whether the study is judged to work or not.

A number of prayer studies chose to measure the clinical outcome of the person being prayed for – whether the person gets better or not. This method is partly historical because the first prayer studies were done that way, and because naturally, if we pray to a deity, we're asking for a person (or ourselves) to be made well. For example, we usually ask 'Please, God, make John well.' We don't say 'Please, God, as you know, John is suffering with painful arthritis. Please let my positive intentions be registered in his nervous system.'

Many prayer studies that measure clinical outcome are, of course, successful, like the Randolph Byrd study I mentioned in the previous chapter, but some aren't, as the Cochrane review pointed out. Some psi researchers say that it's very difficult to effectively control for a clinical outcome because it can be affected by other things.

So, in many of the more recent studies, rather than looking for a clinical outcome, the researchers measured whether praying for someone impacts their mental, emotional, or spiritual well-being or the activity in their autonomic nervous system (ANS), which would have a bearing on their recovery.

A More Subtle Approach

Over a span of five years at the Royal Adelaide Hospital Cancer Centre in Australia, 999 cancer patients were prayed for.[9] Rather than looking for a physical health outcome in the patients, though, the researchers decided to measure if the prayer had any effect on their emotional and spiritual well-being. They asked an external group offering prayer to add the patients to their usual prayer lists and gave them a small amount of information about each person. The latter was to facilitate some sense of felt connection.

Over the course of the study, there were significantly greater improvements in both spiritual and emotional well-being compared with a similar-sized group who weren't prayed for.

And a randomized controlled trial published in 2020 found that being prayed for improved the coping ability and spiritual well-being of women receiving radiotherapy for breast cancer.[10] Prayers were offered by a group who asked for calm, peace, harmony, and recovery of health and spiritual well-being. All the patients had asked for prayers, but only half were actually prayed for, and only in those women were improvements seen in coping and spiritual well-being.

One advantage of measuring an effect on the ANS is that it's affected by a person's state of consciousness. So, if the consciousness of one person is able to impact on the consciousness of another, which the consciousness equation (*see page 184*) predicts, then this may well show up in the person's ANS and researchers can obtain a physical, objective measure of the impact of consciousness.

And another advantage of ANS studies is that they can be done under more controlled conditions in a laboratory. If studies try to measure only clinical outcomes, there are many other factors that can impact the result, but measuring the ANS response of a person while they're being prayed for leaves much less to chance. In addition, ANS studies show whether there's an absolute effect or not.

Clinical outcome studies can miss an effect because they're looking for something more significant, such as how fast a person recovered, or how many side effects they had from their treatment, or how many painkillers they took – not whether an effect exists or not. An effect might be registered in the ANS, for example, but it might be missed when measuring a broader clinical outcome.

And if the impact of consciousness is generally small in these types of studies, then we need to be looking for small effects. As I said earlier, in psi work we don't typically test for whether a person can move a pencil across a desk with their mind, but for more subtle effects, so we choose measurements that are of the right level of sensitivity. We need to use scales of measurement that are appropriate to the size of the effect being measured.

It would be ludicrous to try to measure gravitational waves using a 12-inch (30-cm) ruler, for example. The sensitivity of the LIGO experiment that first detected gravitational waves, a prediction of Einstein's general theory of relativity, was equivalent to measuring the width of the Atlantic Ocean to within the thickness of an atom (or equivalent to measuring the distance to the nearest star with an accuracy of the thickness of a human hair). Similarly, we don't try to measure the strong nuclear force between subatomic particles by measuring the attraction between two apples or oranges.

As I said earlier, in my experience, part of the skepticism around psi stems from the assumption that if mind impacts matter, then we should all be mentally willing objects (and ourselves) to levitate. Since that tends not to happen, skeptics deduce that the entire phenomenon is false. Measurements in psi experiments, as they are in other fields of science, need to be appropriate to the scale of the phenomena being measured.

CHAPTER 11

The Law of Attraction

At the University of British Columbia in Vancouver, Canada, more than 200 female students were told that in mathematics, boys typically score 5 percentile points higher than girls.[1] It wasn't actually true.

Half of the girls were told that the difference in achievement was related to a gene on the Y chromosome, which only males have, which causes an increase in energy supply to a region of the brain involved in focusing on mental tasks. The other half were told it was down to stereotyping – believing that boys do better than girls, parents and teachers bias their expectations from early school years and treat boys and girls differently.

When they sat a math test sometime later, the girls who believed the difference in achievement between boys and girls was due to stereotyping significantly outperformed those who believed they were at a genetic disadvantage. Each girl's performance in math came down to what she *believed*.

At the University of Wisconsin, a study of 30,000 people found that the *perception* that stress is bad for one's health is arguably worse than stress itself, ranking as the 15th leading cause of death in the USA, just behind hypertension and hypertensive renal disease (13th), and Parkinson's disease (14th).[2]

Being highly stressed and believing it's bad for you increased the risk of early death by 43 percent when compared to having the same amount of stress but perceiving it's good for you. In the same study, the death rate among one group of people who experienced only a small amount of stress was higher than it was among a group of people who were highly stressed. Again, the reason was that the low-stress group *believed* that stress was bad for them while the high stress group believed that stress was good for them.

Beyond math scores and health, much of life is influenced by our beliefs. A person who believes they're a failure sees obstacles as insurmountable problems, whereas someone who believes that they're successful tackles problems head on as they arise, with the attitude that they can be solved. If these two people meet the same challenge at the same time, whether they succeed or fail isn't necessarily determined by individual ability but by what they each believe about themselves.

> *Our beliefs shape our experiences to a very large degree. If you believe you can do something you'll usually fare better than if you believe you can't.*

You're more likely to try in the first place, more likely to spot solutions, and more likely to go the extra mile if it's necessary.

In his book *Wishes Fulfilled: Mastering the Art of Manifesting*, Dr. Wayne Dyer wrote, 'If you believe it will work out, you'll see opportunities. If you believe it won't, you will see obstacles.'[3]

In one sense, our beliefs impact our lives akin to the way they impact our brain chemistry; in both cases, life – whether as circumstances or brain chemistry – meets our expectations. And if it happens to be true that matter is how consciousness appears, then we might expect this.

The Butterfly Effect

In the branch of mathematics known as chaos theory, the butterfly effect is the 'sensitive dependence on initial conditions.' It's where a small change in one state can result in large changes further down the line. It's popularly known by the metaphor of a butterfly flapping its wings in one place and causing a tornado thousands of miles away a few weeks later. But aspects of the butterfly effect apply in our lives all the time.

Let's say you leave the house for work one day but forget your car keys and have to return to get them. The extra few minutes this takes delays your arrival on the highway, which results in your getting stuck in traffic because there's been an accident that you'd have been ahead of if you hadn't forgotten your keys.

The knock-on effect of arriving late at work is missing an important meeting that may have landed you a big sales deal and possibly even a promotion as a result. Thus, your hoped-for bonus and salary increase fail to materialize, so you're unable to buy that bigger house with more space for your family, or take them on that holiday you'd all been dreaming of. In this instance of the 'sensitive dependence on initial conditions,' everything escalated from you forgetting your car keys.

I think most of us have had a similar experience to this, in which a seemingly small and insignificant action had far-reaching consequences; we've probably also seen how a small misunderstanding can escalate into something quite major.

The other side of the butterfly effect is that seemingly small *positive* things can escalate too. Forgetting your car keys might have helped you to avoid that accident, or meant that you ended up meeting someone who had become very important in your life – an opportunity you'd have missed if you hadn't returned home to get your keys. The sensitive dependence on initial conditions also means that seemingly improbable things can happen, even from just a small action.

Paddling the River of Life

Many people today talk of using the law of attraction to attract what they want. Essentially, this 'universal law,' which was popularized in the documentary *The Secret* and the best-selling book by Rhonda Byrne that followed it, states that we'll attract into our lives whatever we focus on. In this sense, the belief is that our state or consciousness seems to attract the objects or events that we're focusing on.

The word attract, as it's used here, doesn't necessarily mean that the subject of your focus will literally fall out of the sky and land on your lap, in the way a magnet attracts a piece of iron – it simply means that you and that which you focus on tend to come together in some way.

The law of attraction as it's generally understood can be misleading though. It suggests that if you think positive then only positive things will happen. Although this notion is potentially inspiring and can fill some people with hope, it can also be quite upsetting to individuals who are experiencing difficult life situations, who rightly point out that bad things do indeed happen to good people.

To my understanding, it's not quite so plain and straightforward as positive thoughts produce positive things. However, I do believe that having consistently positive thoughts produces a general movement in that direction, and that even when bad things happen, our attitude and thinking can help us navigate a course through them.

I think of it as like being in a canoe on a wide river. We have a paddle, which means we can paddle to the left or right, or even around in a circle if we prefer. The idea that we attract what we focus on is like using our paddle to get to where we want to go. The paddle represents our thinking and actions.

But what we sometimes miss is that the river has a current. Sometimes it's very gentle and it seems as if life flows easily, and that we do seem to effortlessly attract what we focus on. Other times the current is relatively calm but there are little eddies that knock us off direction; however, with some clear focus and steady, consistent paddling, we still reach our intended destination.

On occasion, there's a strong current pulling us in the opposite direction from where we're trying to go. And there are times in our lives when, let's be honest, we're in the rapids and it seems that no amount of positive thought is working. And we hit the rocks head-on! Spiritual teachers advise that during such times we should 'let go,' or 'go with the flow' – they say we should trust that we're where we need to be and that we'll get to where we need to go, and turn our thoughts to acceptance.

It seems to me that in life in general, outside of the rapids, adopting a consistently positive attitude can gradually influence our direction, as if we're making steady, consistent paddling movements toward where we want to go.

Paddling is a metaphor not only for attitude but also for taking physical action – sometimes to propel ourselves in the direction of our hopes and dreams, and other times to push forward and counteract challenges and setbacks. For example, a person who puts their dreams and attitudes into action by taking consistently positive action will almost always fare better than someone who visualizes a dream and then twiddles their thumbs as they wait for it to show up.

Taking Consistent Action

I was discussing the law of attraction with an acquaintance when he enthusiastically declared: 'You had a dream to be a published author. Now look at you. You totally attracted that!' And he was right. If you look at my starting mindset and the eventual outcome, that's exactly what happened.

I visualized having a book published and believed I could do it. I eventually came together with the object of my focus. However, there was a long period between wish and outcome that necessitated consistent action on my part.

I started writing my first book in 1998, on one Sunday morning in a coffee shop in an English town where I worked locally for a pharmaceutical company. I discarded what I'd written a few months later and, over the next few years, I started writing and then discarding what I'd written on two more occasions.

My fourth attempt began at the end of January 2003, three years after I'd left the pharmaceutical industry. At the time, I had two part-time teaching jobs, one as a lecturer in chemistry at a college outside Glasgow in Scotland, and the other as a chemistry tutor in the Department of Adult and Continuing Education at Glasgow University. For early classes I'd take a bus at 5:45 a.m. and sometimes I wouldn't get home until after 11 p.m.

Given my travel and teaching commitments, it was very difficult to find time to follow my dream of writing a book. But it was important to me. I realized that the only way I could do it was to write through the night a few times a week. My first class started at 1 p.m. on three days a week, so I wrote from around midnight until 3 a.m. four times a week (once on the weekend) and had a lie-in before traveling to class. I did this for about six months to produce the first draft of the book. It then took another 18 months to shape it into the final version.

When it was finally complete, my book, *It's the Thought That Counts*, was rejected by every publisher I sent it to. So I self-published it in May 2005, seven years after I'd started writing it. Hay House UK republished it the following October. Ultimately, I'd 'manifested' my desire. I'd 'attracted' what I wanted. It just took a heck of a lot of perseverance and legwork along the way.

Reid Tracy, President and CEO of Hay House Publishers, once told me, 'It takes 10 years to be an overnight success.' We'd been talking about people's perception of success and the prevailing belief that successful people simply have a thought, take a few actions, and boom – dream fulfilled. But they don't always realize that there's a bit in between that quite often requires focus, dedication, sweat, tears, and a fair bit of consistent action.

Nudging Life's Chemistry

While he was at the top of the world of soccer, David Beckham was considered one of the best ever free-kick takers. People called it natural talent, and that was definitely a factor, but what most didn't know about was his work ethic. At the end of training sessions, when the other players had gone home to their families or out with friends, Beckham would still be on the pitch, kicking ball after ball, practicing hundreds and hundreds of free kicks to hone his talent; and he did that for years.

Carl Lewis, considered one of the greatest athletes of all time, frequently stayed behind at the track after training, making jump after jump after jump for hours until he got it just right. He became one of the most technically gifted long jumpers ever. But it was practice that got him there.

Many top athletes use visualization as well as practice. You may recall the examples I shared in Chapter 1 of Ed Moses and Sally Gunnell, who used repetitive visualization to help them achieve their goals. They combined visualization with consistent *action*.

> *Consistent action helps us attract*
> *what we want in life.*

Of course, given what I've written in the past three chapters, there must also be an influence from our state of consciousness. Even though it's not been formally studied in science, I suspect that holding a consistent mental vision of what we want must, to some degree, influence the circumstances and conditions in our lives. That is, of course, if we continue with the assumption that consciousness isn't locked inside the skull, which I'm clearly making here.

It may be that in between our actions, some seemingly strange coincidences and synchronicities occur as the amount of our consciousness that we point toward something nudges the chemistry of life, as it does the chemistry of the brain when we believe something.

And by the chemistry of life, I mean events, circumstances, and what other people say and do. If conscious intention can impact another person's consciousness and nervous system at a distance, move an arrow on a screen, and create patterns in random numbers, it seems to me that it's quite likely that our minds nudge the chemistry of our lives in seemingly invisible ways.

Small Things Accumulate

While summarizing the research that took place at the PEAR laboratory of Princeton University – which investigated interactions of human consciousness with devices called RNGs (random number generators) – Roger Nelson, who had coordinated much of the research, wrote, 'Over more than a decade, this basic experiment yielded an enormous database, with a bottom line indicating a small but significant effect of human intention on random data sequences.'[4] As I explained in Chapter 9, the effect size was small on average; it wasn't of the size of levitating objects, but it was there all the same, and it was real. What does it mean in real life?

Nelson was referring to the random data produced by a computer. As far as those experiments went, human consciousness created small, statistically significant patterns in the numbers. Consciousness impacted a physical system.

To my mind, this suggests that consciousness isn't inside the head, and that idealism or some form of it, or panpsychism, or some form of it, or something in between the two, offers a more accurate description of the world than does materialism. Perhaps matter is an appearance of consciousness (idealism) but all matter has experience (panpsychism).

It means that a person's consciousness can influence things in the physical world. The effect might be small – we're not talking about having the powers of Wonder Woman or the X-Men – but given the sensitive dependence on initial conditions, small effects may turn out to be meaningful, especially if conscious intention supplies a steady and consistent paddling direction on our metaphorical river – that is, if we hold an image in our minds of what we want or where we want to get to.

Small things accumulate. If you add up a lot of small effects that occur in each moment, after a number of moments you can end up with something big that's noticeable; it's like making the occasional tiny movement of the paddle to the right and after several miles of water, realizing that you've reached the right bank. But that's *only* the case if you maintain your focus, which many of us don't.

The Importance of Holding Our Focus

I've fond memories of playing with my sisters in the back garden of my granny and papa's house when I was a young child. Sometimes in the summer, the garden hose would lie on the grass, and my papa or Uncle Daniel would turn the tap on full. The hose would rise into the air like a snake, and then make random movements all over the place as the force of the water coursed through it. My sisters and I would laugh as we each darted in and out, making futile attempts to take control of the hose.

In the years since, I've come to realize that most people's minds are like that hose, darting one way and then the next, not holding for long in any one direction.

> *Sometimes, we don't attract the things*
> *we want in life because we fail to*
> *maintain a consistent focus on them.*

We chop and change, going from wishing to achieve something to thinking it's not possible, to wishing it again and then doubting ourselves once more, to eventually forgetting about it altogether, only to think about it again several years later and lament that we never achieved it.

Can Our Consciousness Influence Our Lives?

If you knew, or at least believed a little, that the focus of your consciousness could influence the circumstances and conditions in your life, would you allow yourself to dream more and hold your focus more consistently?

Suppose I'm waiting for a mail delivery one day, and in each moment that I wait there are multiple events happening in my environment – in that of the postal worker and in that of each person who interacts with her, now and in the time period before the delivery of my package. The question I'd like to pose is, given that consciousness impacts people and things, could the focus of my consciousness impact the postal worker and other people in the environment and influence when my delivery arrives?

It may seem woo-woo even to contemplate such a question, but if our consciousnesses do impact each other, then some of the influence may be just enough to nudge the timing of events. So, I'd respond in the affirmative to this question, and go so far as to say that we're doing this kind of thing all the time in our lives, as Donald Hoffman, creator of the interface theory of perception, maintains. We're affecting others and we're being affected by others in subtle ways.

In the latter sense, we're unknowingly participating in others' experience of attracting the things they want. We just don't notice all this because we're not really paying much attention to the content of our mind, and when seemingly coincidental things happen we're so conditioned in our materialist mindset that we write them off as chance.

But what if they're not chance? What if it's not *just a coincidence* that a person you were thinking about suddenly contacts you, and that you actually sensed their conscious intention to contact you or that your thought prompted them to contact you, or both?

> *What if we really do influence things,*
> *perhaps some things only a little,*
> *but others maybe much more?*

Let's return to our postal delivery example. At one point, the driver stops the vehicle, picks up some packages, and steps out. She has to look left and right to cross the road as there are a few vehicles passing. She walks to another house in the road where I live and knocks on the door. She waits until the person answers the door and they have a short, friendly verbal exchange. She then walks along the road and knocks on another couple of doors, and enjoys similar exchanges, before eventually arriving at my home.

Think of all the micro events that are taking place in any instant in this scenario – the movement of traffic; the feet of the drivers on the pedals; people's interior environments and the conversations and happenings inside their homes that affect their choices and determine *when* they open the door; the nature and content of the conversations the postal worker has with each person who opens their door, and much more.

Would my consciousness influence some of these things in ways that are small but could escalate? Maybe it causes small changes in a conversation with a neighbor, or a slight, seemingly unconscious increase or decrease in the walking pace of the postal worker. And this might just be enough to escalate into my package arriving a few seconds (or minutes) earlier or later.

Let's say I'm doing something important that I need to finish before the knock at the door interrupts me. Perhaps I have a strong faith and feel a connection with God, so I offer a short prayer to that effect. Or I strongly imagine just making it in time and I feel a relaxed sense of absorption in that moment. Might the focus of my consciousness subtly impact enough of these micro events and somehow slow the delivery person?

Not Just a Coincidence

I appreciate how unlikely this sounds, especially to people who aren't used to considering such ideas, but if the research presented in the previous chapters is valid, then it might be possible.

As I said, I think we're doing this sort of thing all the time – as the influencer and influencee – but we largely don't notice it or we dismiss it as chance. How many times do we say after something happens, 'I was just thinking about that yesterday,' and then write it off as a coincidence? It may often be that you influenced it happening, or intuited the likelihood of it.

If the effect size of our consciousnesses impacting on each other happens to be around the same magnitude as when we influence the random data of an RNG, then it seems logical that we do influence our personal realities to an extent when we wish for something to happen, and especially if we feel a sense of absorption or connection.

And sometimes, when the conditions are right and not the 'cold' conditions of a testing lab, we might give our personal reality a bit more of a push, exerting a considerably greater force of consciousness on it.

Feeling What We Want

We can relate the consciousness equation we explored in Chapter 8 to the law of attraction. In this context, the amount of consciousness is the amount of your consciousness focused upon your wish, hope, dream, or belief, and the distance in consciousness represents your felt connection with your wish, hope, dream or belief – the object of your focus.

When I spoke of fields of consciousness earlier, the 'felt connection' I outlined was between you and the wholeness of consciousness, the universe, or God, but it can really be a felt connection with anything. It can be the object of your focus – just as the people who were most successful at influencing the RNGs were those who felt a sense of absorption with the machine or experiment.

So, to seemingly attract something you want into your life, as well as holding a consistent focus on it, it might help to *feel* it – to imagine the thing as if it's already happened and allow yourself to feel good about it. The consciousness equation would predict that this would cause a stronger interaction between you and the object of your focus, and so you'd be more likely to draw it to yourself and you to it.

Again, let me reiterate that I'm not speaking of the object of your desire flying through the air and landing on your lap, but of a subtle but steady organizing of events and circumstances in the direction of what you're focusing on, in such a way that can sometimes produce surprising outcomes.

This is precisely what some proponents of the law of attraction suggest – that we think of the thing we want as if it has already happened, and allow ourselves to feel it as if it's so. For example, in *Feeling is the Secret*, author and mystic Neville Goddard writes: 'Call your desires into being by imagining and feeling your wish fulfilled.'

And What We Don't Want

Felt connection matters, but often our dominant felt connection is in the opposite direction of what we want, so this can make it *appear* as if we don't attract what we want at all. As an example, let's say you want a new car. That's your desire. But say your dominant focus is not on the new car but on how much you hate your present car – how much it costs you, how often it breaks down, the scrapes and rust, and so on.

Your present car annoys you so much that rather than dreaming about how great it would be to have the new car, you dwell more on feeling frustrated at your present condition. And you spend more time talking to people about the issues you have with your current car than about what kind of car you'd actually like and how amazing it would be to have it.

In this instance, where is your felt connection and amount of consciousness pointed? To the issues with your current car – so *that's* what you're attracting: more time and more issues with your current car. Of this type of experience, Dr. Wayne Dyer offered, 'Perhaps the most common misuse of imagination is stressing what you don't want for yourself.'

Navigating the Waves

Before I go further with these ideas, let me be clear that this doesn't mean it's a person's fault when bad things happen. For example, no one attracts the death of a loved one because they were thinking negative thoughts for a while. No one attracts being in a place of famine. Negative thinking didn't get them there and positive thinking might do little to get them out of it.

The playing fields of life aren't level. Some people's circumstances make it easier for them to focus on what they want and believe they can achieve it, whereas other people's make doing so extremely difficult, given the weight of the challenges in their lives.

A person who is popular and has many friends might focus on attracting a soulmate, but another who is in an abusive relationship is focused on survival. While the goal of a person who lives in a relatively affluent society might be to have a million dollars, for a mother who lives in poverty in a famine-ridden country, the immediate goal is a morsel of food for her children.

> **Much of life is about how we deal with events when they occur, not just about what we're trying to attract.**

When something seemingly bad happens in a person's life, they might sometimes be able to correlate it with the general pattern of thinking that led up to it; but they might not, because it may have occurred for another reason entirely.

We can think of our conscious intentions as waves going outward. But you're not the only person creating waves. While you focus on your hopes and dreams, you rise and fall on the waves created by others, some of which are small and some of which are large. It's not just about you.

The challenge is often in navigating the waves of life while at the same time focusing on your hopes and dreams. Some people find it easier than others to get through difficult times or to maintain a focus on their goals.

Some people are very resilient – they have strong sails. Others become more frustrated about things, sometimes because that way of being is natural for them and sometimes because their life experience has provided them with so many difficult circumstances, they've felt more or less powerless against the seeming weight of life.

It's easy to feel powerful when life is flowing for you, but it's equally easy to feel powerless when your dominant life experience is one of overwhelm or of having little control. I think we all know what both are like from personal experience at particular times in our lives.

But hope lies in the fact that we can improve our mental skills with practice, just as one can learn to play the piano or become a better tennis player. Given the message throughout this book, mental practice might be one of the most important things you ever do. Practice maintaining calm when things seem chaotic. Practice holding your focus on what you want – even when reality is showing you something different or when people around you are critical.

Practice being kind, even when others aren't. Meditation can help with all this. Even against the backdrop of circumstances, mental practice can help you paint the kind of picture you want of your life.

Magical Thinking and the Consciousness Constant

Perhaps with enough practice of focus and belief, and given enough time, seemingly magical things can happen in our lives. Personally, I've experienced some remarkable happenings that I felt could only be attributed to some form of interaction between my consciousness and my physical reality.

Years ago while on a day trip, I urgently needed some floppy disks. I pulled into a large but empty car park in the middle of nowhere, which must have contained more than 100 spaces, and as I stepped out of the car I discovered a box of floppy disks sitting right in the center of the adjacent space, still in their cellophane wrapping.

Having heard numerous similar stories from other people, I've noticed that these kinds of experiences tend to happen more frequently when we entertain the idea that our consciousness interacts with reality. Here, there's a greater amount of our consciousness accepting it – believing in the notion.

According to the consciousness equation, we might therefore experience more of a seeming conscious interaction with our reality. It doesn't mean that if you believe that your consciousness shapes your reality everything you want will land in your lap. As I've said a few times already, I think we're all secretly hoping that the power of our consciousness is enough to help us manifest objects out of thin air, like in the movies.

I'd like to draw your attention once more to the constant C in the consciousness equation, which we discussed in the 'consciousness constant' section in Chapter 9 (*see page 216*). I hypothesized that this does something similar to the Universal Gravitational Constant, G, which is a 'damping' constant.

As I explained, the effect of a damping constant is a reduction in the magnitude of something. I pointed out that if the Universal Gravitational Constant didn't have the value it has, gravity would squash us as flat as a pancake.

If it's true that the contents of our consciousness do attract circumstances to us, then the damping constant would reduce the magnitude of the effect. Rather than pushing, pulling, and levitating people, objects, and events, we'd exert a very subtle effect. As a result, most of the time we'd observe a sort of time lag between thought and reality, where we generally need a consistent, repetitive focus on what we want to best shape things.

But the same also applies to stuff you *don't* want. You have to give those things consistent focus too, which I accept many of us already do. But with awareness of the process, we can learn to move toward the things and experiences we want, and have enough time to catch ourselves if our dominant focus is taking us on a route toward a negative experience.

If there wasn't some damping effect of consciousness, while our imagination might create wonders in our lives, I think many of us would also create nightmares. And I'm not sure there are many people on the planet who, when faced with a nightmare – even if they thought it was of their own creation – would simply be able to think it away. It therefore generally takes repetition, over time, of the same kind of thought or intention to attract something we want.

There's a skill to becoming aware of the contents of your own mind – to realizing what your dominant thinking is about certain things and learning to recognize your beliefs (about yourself, others, and the world) and what you think is and isn't possible for you.

Are there Different Types of Consciousness?

Since I formulated the consciousness equation I've often pondered on the damping constant. I've wondered if it takes different values – sometimes more, sometimes less. Perhaps it is what it is for humans but it's different for other species. As I've explained, I make no secret of the fact that I believe that either idealism or panpsychism offer a more accurate picture of the world than materialism.

> *I believe that consciousness is*
> *fundamental. So we humans can't be*
> *the only 'things' with consciousness.*

We also can't therefore claim to be the only species to attract the contents of their consciousness. I've also wondered about different types of consciousness. As I said earlier, and this is consistent with many spiritual writings, at the moment of complete felt connection with the universe, we essentially *become* the universe in our conscious experience.

The consciousness equation suggests that there are different degrees of magnitude of consciousness that relate to the different degrees of felt connection or different degrees of 'dissociation from the single consciousness,' to borrow Bernardo Kastrup's term. Perhaps there are different quanta of dissociation, like levels or rungs on a ladder, and each quanta, or level, relates to a different value of the consciousness constant. Ours produces a large suppressing effect, so there's a time lag between conscious intention and the manifestation of it.

But perhaps there are other consciousnesses, even those we call angels, that are aspects of the infinite consciousness and are merely a bit less dissociated than we humans. For them, the magnitude of the damping effect may be much less. The contents of their consciousness would manifest much more quickly, perhaps with no time lag at all.

Of course, this is all conjecture. But as I near the end of the book, I thought it might be nice to speculate freely and share with readers some of the contents of my consciousness.

Synchronicity

I've enjoyed numerous discussions with well-educated people about the idea that consciousness can influence reality. In these, we've considered those strange coincidences that appeared to coincide with what we'd been thinking of at the time, and whether or not our states of consciousness had influenced them. In general, some of those people maintained that coincidences happen all the time – which again, I feel stems from a lifelong habit of belief that consciousness is created by the brain and is therefore locked inside the skull.

The assumption is that seemingly non-ordinary coincidences are statistically likely in any large enough population, so there will always be, as one of those people said, 'statistical correlations between non-connected things in any one day.' And of course, that *is* correct. There *will* be such correlations, but that needn't mean there aren't real and meaningful connections at least some of the time.

For example, have you ever suddenly thought about someone you haven't seen in a while and then bumped into them a few days later? Many explain away such instances as coincidence and circumstance, but I believe that they're not.

Carl Jung, the highly influential Swiss psychiatrist and psychoanalyst, wrote that events (and people) are connected through meaning (consciousness) as well as by causality.[5] In other words, some events are more than just one thing appearing to cause another thing and are more deeply connected, such that the seemingly causal connection was always likely to manifest.

He said that some seemingly unconnected events (and people) literally 'fall together' in time and that it's the connection between them that actually *causes* their co-incidence – that is, their happening together at the same time. He called them synchronicities.

Colleagues of Wolfgang Pauli, one of the most brilliant physicists of the 20th century, noted that sensitive technical equipment would incur critical failure whenever he entered a laboratory. The phenomenon happened so frequently that it became affectionately known among physicists as the Pauli Effect.

Pauli is best known for the Pauli Exclusion Principle, for which he received the Nobel Prize for Physics. It's a quantum mechanical principle that states that no two fermions (a class of subatomic particle) can occupy the same quantum state at the same time. Colleagues joked that Pauli and any functioning piece of equipment could also not occupy the same room at the same time and called this the 'second' Pauli Exclusion Principle.

Pauli and Jung were good friends and shared similar ideas around synchronicity. Through his own personal observations and discussions with Jung, Pauli came to believe that the Pauli Effect was indeed real.[6]

The theoretical physicist and renowned cosmologist George Gamow wrote about a synchronicity that concerned Pauli in his 1966 book *Thirty Years That Shook Physics: The Story of Quantum Theory.*[7] One day in the laboratory of Nobel Prize-winning physicist James Franck in Göttingen, Germany, a piece of complicated and sensitive experimental equipment for studying atoms broke down for no apparent reason.

Franck and his colleagues scratched their heads, wondering what could have happened, because there was no logical explanation for it. They joked that the only possible explanation was that Pauli must be around somewhere.

Well, it turned out that they were right. Pauli had been traveling from his home in Zurich, Switzerland, to visit the lab of Niels Bohr in Copenhagen, Denmark. His train had stopped for a few minutes at Göttingen Station at the exact time that Franck's equipment had broken down. Jung and Pauli believed that people and things are far more connected than physical appearances show.

Connections through Time

You may recall the mental image I shared earlier of a 3D web, the strands of which connect all people and all things, with the thicker strands representing people who share an emotional connection. I imagine those strands as made of light, only the light is consciousness.

The web also connects things (people and events) through time. As we move through time and space, certain people and events are drawn together because they have a connection in consciousness, even if there's no logical physical connection (yet) – or as Jung put it, they 'fall together in time.'

> **As mystical as it sounds, the future connection of people and events may be the force that drives some coincidences.**

In fact, evidence from quantum mechanical experiments and from RNG studies by the PEAR group and others suggests that this may indeed be the case. There may therefore be *some* (not all) things that are more or less 'meant' to happen. The synchronistic connection acts like a magnet in the present, pulling people and particular sets of circumstances together, however seemingly improbable at times.

Many events, then, happen not because they've been causally created – although there will seem to be a logical series of events that led to them – but because the real force shaping them was that they were *already* connected. Those involved in these occurrences are simply drawn to make conscious and unconscious choices that result in them happening.

In the present, when we have thoughts, hopes, and dreams, it's as if a pulse of light (consciousness) is sent out into the web, as vibrations through its strands. People who can help us in some way, however small, feel an impulse on a subconscious level. The impulse inspires them to turn left instead of right, or to forget their keys, or to miss the train they were intending to catch, or to take a little longer in a particular shop.

As a result, that day, we have a seemingly chance encounter with someone who turns out to be just the person we needed to meet. We can write these things off as luck or coincidence, or we can accept that there's sometimes a deeper reason for the occurrence.

A Nudge from Another Consciousness

A few years ago, while in the midst of creating a blog for my website about the possible interaction of consciousness with reality, I remembered that I needed to place an order for copies of my own books for a lecture I was giving in a few days' time. I made the call to my publisher's distributer around 11:45 a.m., just before the noon cut-off time.

Afterward, I continued with the blog for an hour or so. I wanted to add a reference from a book about Einstein's relativity theories called *Why Does E = mc²?* by the particle physicists Brian Cox and Jeff Forshaw. I'd read it a year or so earlier, but I realized that my copy was in storage (I was moving house at the time).

In that moment I felt so frustrated because I really wanted to re-familiarize myself with the book and it wasn't possible. Looking upward, with my arms outstretched, I shook my hands vigorously as I beseeched the universe: 'I *really* need that book.' It was done half in jest (this is the sort of light and playful way I relate to the universe/unified consciousness/God, as if it were a friend) and half in clear thinking and determination.

As I completed the wording in the blog, I had the sensation that I'd just described the science behind the 1999 movie *The Matrix*. I felt a strange sense of absorption, as if I'd hit on a profound truth that I hadn't previously realized with as much clarity. I pressed 'post' to upload the blog to my website.

No more than a handful of seconds later, the phone rang and it was my publisher's distributor. A woman in customer services by the name of Michelle informed me that there had been... *wait for it* ... 'a glitch in the system.' (Fans of *The Matrix* will remember the scene where Trinity says, 'A déjà vu is usually a glitch in the Matrix. It happens when they change something.')

Somehow, Michelle explained, the warehouse staff hadn't fulfilled my entire order (of about 100 books) and had instead packed and dispatched a box of just 10 books for delivery the following day. As a result, I wouldn't receive all the books I needed for my lecture. She sincerely apologized, but I assured her it was fine and that she needn't worry about it; I wanted her to know that it wasn't her fault in any way.

The following day, the box of 10 books arrived, and as I opened it, something looked odd. Near the middle of the pile was a book with its spine facing in the opposite direction – it was a single copy of *Why Does E = mc²?!* I stood bolt upright and backed toward the wall. It gave me a fright, to be perfectly honest.

Only once previously, in more than a decade of ordering books almost monthly from that distributor, had I received a 'mispick,' as it's known (they'd sent 25 copies of a children's Christmas book instead of 25 copies of my book *How Your Mind Can Heal Your Body*). But a single copy of the very book for which I'd beseeched the universe inside a pack of my own books?

> **There's statistics and there's statistics, but this stretched the limits of even the most sensible attempt to explain it away with chance or clever mathematics.**

It was an example of synchronicity. Afterward, as I tried to rationalize the experience, I rolled a few thoughts around in my mind. I considered the possibility that my consciousness had sent vibrations through the web of consciousness that had influenced the warehouse staff.

I also contemplated whether I'd experienced a nudge from another consciousness. After all, when a person dies, it's possible that their consciousness dissolves back into the whole, or into a larger aspect of the being we knew them to be, like a wave falling back into the ocean. As far as I'm concerned, they still exist, only in a larger, less dissociated form; in a sense, closer to God, the universe, unified consciousness in their felt experience. Could it have been the consciousness of a grandparent, then, or even of my dog, Oscar, who had passed away a year earlier and to whom I'd been so close?

My Guidance

The experience felt so significant that I decided it was intentional guidance for me. I decided to believe that I was *supposed* to re-read *Why Does E = mc²?* And in a roundabout way, doing so helped me to write *this* book. Let me explain.

At that time, unknown to my family, friends, or publisher, I was feeling lost and was considering giving up my career as a writer and speaker for something that provided more stability. It can be a tough path, especially when most of your income is dependent on securing bookings for speaking events and enough people turning up at them for you to be paid. I was so weary of living from month to month, never knowing if I'd even earn enough to pay the mortgage.

Although many people thought of me as a successful author, due to the relatively small payments I received for many of the talks I did, and the substantial travel and accommodation expenses I incurred, my income was only just above the UK average at the time, and I worked around 60 hours a week to make it. There were times when it cost me more to travel to a speaking event than I'd be paid to speak.

I felt tired and eventually, during one speaking trip, I made a definitive decision to work toward a new career, probably in academia. I felt a sense of relief. I'd just finished reading the copy of *Why Does E = mc²?* that had arrived with my books and intuited that math and physics was the direction in which I had to head.

I arrived home from that trip late on a Sunday night, and as I walked through the door I learned of the death of Dr. Wayne Dyer, a pioneering author and speaker in the field of self-development. Wayne had been a personal hero of mine. When I first left the pharmaceutical industry I listened to recordings of his work on cassette tapes, and these greatly influenced the direction my own writing took and the kind of person I became.

Over the years, listening to Wayne speak became a source of great comfort and inspiration to me, and his passing gave me a jolt. It reminded me how much I love what I do. Despite the financial challenges I felt at that time, I love writing, speaking, and teaching. I'd always wanted to be like Wayne, and I knew I had to continue as a writer and speaker, no matter what. Perhaps moving toward math and physics didn't need to be a career change, I reasoned, but something that would help me to write better books and be a better teacher.

At around the same time, I was also having a recurring dream, a nightmare really, in which I'd reach the end of a school or university term without having completed any of my math assignments. I always woke up in a sweat and feeling anxious, sometimes not sure if I was awake or dreaming, and with the sense that I was supposed to be doing math but was going to run out of time.

The subject matter of Cox and Forshaw's book deeply inspired me; in fact, Einstein's relativity theories lit me up so much that I decided to study them formally. I registered with the Open University in the UK to undertake a part-time degree in mathematics and physics which, at the time of writing this book, I've almost completed. I never had the dream again after I'd registered for the degree.

That nudge from another consciousness, as I interpreted it, led me to immerse myself more fully in mathematics and physics, and Wayne's passing around the same time ultimately guided me back to where I needed to be as a writer and speaker. Writing this book has felt like stretching a muscle to become more flexible, only it was *me* who was stretching. As I found myself stretching further in my understanding of science, I found a counterbalance in simultaneously stretching further in my spiritual experience of life. It's this two-way stretch that enabled me to create this fusion of science and spirituality.

Conclusion

My intention when I began this book was to gather the scientific evidence where it exists for those subjects that are so often unfairly dismissed as pseudoscience or airy-fairy mysticism, and where it didn't, to at least provide a basis in science or philosophy for why something *might* be true.

In so doing, I hoped I could reduce some of the knee-jerk skepticism that surrounds meditation, reiki, crystals, and other complementary therapies, because a lot of people enjoy them and I believe they should be able to practice them without judgment.

As I've said, this skepticism often stems from the fact that the scientific research that supports many of these practices is little known by the general public. So, I hope I've now provided enough of that. I've personally witnessed how beneficial complementary approaches to health and well-being can be. While some people clearly require medical interventions, many would gain much from a practice that treats and restores the whole person, which is something that complementary therapies can provide.

This is why I've suggested that, given the increasing use of complementary practices and their inclusion in large hospitals around the world, we should continue with a closer integration between complementary and conventional medicine.

It needn't be one or the other, but both. Sometimes, more of one and less of the other, depending on the circumstances; sometimes all of one and none of the other, depending on the circumstances. But a happy fusion of these two seemingly separate worlds appears to be the way forward that will provide the most benefit to patients.

*****

As for the more esoteric subjects covered in this book, among them prayer, distant healing, presentiment (intuition), telepathy, and the law of attraction, the reality of these may rest on consciousness not being locked inside the brain and produced by neurons, but something more fundamental, something universally present.

Certainly, there's been a lot of philosophical thought on this matter stretching back centuries, but solving the 'hard problem of consciousness' is gaining traction in modern times because many have arrived at the conclusion that, while it's been incredibly useful for developing modern technology, the prevailing materialist view can't help us with much of the softer side of life – that of human interaction, of love, of our deeper felt connections with nature that so many of us intuit.

And there's been a great deal of science in support of these connections that we seemingly share, which must exist at the level of our consciousness.

I've presented a mere fraction of the work in the general parapsychology field, which formally studies psi phenomena; there's much, much more, and many books on the subject. Those by Dean Radin are a good place to find much of it collected together. I used some of Dean's books, including *Real Magic* and *Entangled Minds*, as the basis for some of the sections in this book, and then read the papers to which he referred.

Larry Dossey's excellent *Prayer Is Good Medicine* and *The Power of Premonitions* are good resources too, along with Lynne McTaggart's *The Field* and *The Intention Experiment*, and the titles by Rupert Sheldrake I refer to in Chapter 9.

As I've said, the researchers who carry out the studies in these areas show great courage in the face of skepticism and ridicule. I believe that things are shifting, though. The placebo effect and meditation, once regarded with huge skepticism and derided as psychobabble, are now accepted by the scientific mainstream as having many benefits, and the same is happening with visualization.

And as more science accumulates for them, I'm also seeing the same movement in the seemingly more subtle and esoteric fields. I don't know when, or if, psi and other phenomena will enter the mainstream, but there's a definite move in the direction of embracing them more, and this is thanks to those who so diligently carry out the research, and to those who write about it in popular books and magazine articles.

*****

I have to admit that amid those times when I felt most excited and inspired by the content of this book, I also experienced periods of anxiety while writing about it. My last four books, which were my most successful to date, focused on the mind–body connection, self-esteem, and kindness, all of which have moved into the mainstream as more science has became available.

Many professionals and researchers have viewed me with respect for helping to popularize these subjects by offering a scientific basis for them – in particular, the way kindness impacts mental and physical health, and the fact that it's highly contagious, which I explored in *The Five Side Effects of Kindness* and *The Little Book of Kindness*.

But at least half of this book signals quite a departure in subject matter for me, and I've wondered how it will be received by peers who have come to respect my work, as well as by the general reader.

Although I've presented the science and the best available thought, even adding the beginnings of my own mathematical formalism of consciousness interactions – my reason for doing so is that ideas tend to be better accepted when there's a mathematical basis – there's still enough of an air of woo-woo to cause some concern. Will I lose my credibility? Will I be criticized? These have been my main concerns, although I remain confident that the scientific evidence I've presented is sound.

I hope that you've enjoyed the book and have found it interesting and helpful – even if it just provides some scientific confirmation of the things you've always believed. And if you're a therapist or a complementary practitioner, or simply someone who has always had an interest in these things, I hope that it even helps those around you who might previously have been skeptical to better understand how you think, what you do, and why you do it.

References

Introduction

1. Oxford Online Dictionary, https://en.oxforddictionaries.com/definition/woo-woo [Accessed May 11, 2021]

Chapter 1: Mind Over Matter

1. Levine, J.D., et al. (1978), 'The mechanism of placebo analgesia,' *The Lancet*, 312(8091), pp.654–657.

2. Zubieta, J-K., et al. (2005), 'Placebo effects mediated by endogenous opioid activity on μ-opioid receptors,' *The Journal of Neuroscience*, 25(34), pp.7754–7762.

3. Benedetti, F., et al. (2007), 'Opioid mediated placebo responses boost pain endurance and physical performance: is it doping in sport competitions?' *The Journal of Neuroscience*, 27(44), pp.11934–11939.

4. Luparello, T., et al. (1968), 'Influences of suggestion on airway reactivity in asthmatic subjects,' *Psychosomatic Medicine*, 30(6), pp.819–825.

5. Blackwell, B., et al. (1972), 'Demonstration to medical students of placebo responses and non-drug factors,' *The Lancet*, 299(7763), pp.1279–1282.

6. Moerman, D. (2002), *Meaning, Medicine and the 'Placebo Effect.'* Cambridge University Press.

7. De Craen, A.J., et al. (2000), 'Placebo effect in the acute treatment of migraine: Subcutaneous placebos are better than oral placebos,' *Journal of Neurology*, 247(3), pp.183–188.

8. Lambert, R., et al. (1977), 'Treatment of duodenal and gastric ulcer with cimetidine: A multicenter double-blind trial,' *Gastroenterologie Clinique et Biologique*, 1(11), pp.855–860.

9. Branthwaite, A. and Cooper, P. (1981), 'Analgesic effects of branding in treatment of headaches,' *British Medical Journal*, 282, pp.1576–1578.

10. Vallance, A.K. (2006), 'Something out of nothing: the placebo effect,' *Advances in Psychiatric Treatment*, 12, pp.287–296.

11. Thomas, K.B. (1987), 'General practice consultations: is there any point in being positive?' *British Medical Journal*, 294(6581), pp.1200–1202.

12. De la Fuente-Fernández, R., et al. (2001), 'Expectation and dopamine release: mechanism of the placebo effect in Parkinson's disease,' *Science*, 293(5532), pp.1164–1166.

13. Rief, W., et al. (2017), 'Preoperative optimization of patient expectations improves long-term outcome in heart surgery patients: results of the randomized controlled PSY-HEART trial,' *BMC Medicine*, 15(4), pp.1–13.

14. Benedetti, F., et al. (2016), 'Teaching neurons to respond to placebos,' *Journal of Physiology*, 594(19), pp.5647–5660.

15. Goebel, M.U., et al. (2002), 'Behavioral conditioning of immunosuppression is possible in humans,' *FASEB*, 16(14), pp.1869–1873.

16. Sandler, A.D. (2010), 'Conditioned placebo dose reduction: a new treatment in attention-deficit hyperactivity disorder,' *Journal of Developmental and Behavioural Pediatrics*, 31(5), pp.369–375.

17. Mitsikostas, D.D., et al. (2014), 'Nocebo in clinical trials for depression: a meta-analysis,' *Psychiatry Research*, 215(1), pp.82–86.

18. Greener, M. (2018), 'Placebo: a clinical, biological and ethical enigma,' *Independent Nurse*, December, pp.28–31.

19. Weihrauch, T.R. and Gauler, T.C. (1999), 'Placebo – Efficacy and Adverse Effects in Controlled Clinical Trials,' *Arzneimittelforschung*, 49(05), pp.385–393.

20. Pascual-Leone, A. (1995), 'Modulation of muscle responses evoked by transcranial magnetic stimulation during the acquisition of new fine motor skills,' *Journal of Neurophysiology*, 74(3), pp.1037–1045.

21. Ranganathan, V.K., et al. (2004), 'From mental power to muscle power—gaining strength by using the mind,' *Neuropsychologia*, 42(7), pp.944–956.

22. Page, S.J., et al. (2007), 'Mental Practice in Chronic Stroke,' *Stroke*, 38(4), pp.1293–1297.

23. Kho, A.Y. (2013), 'Meta-analysis on the effect of mental imagery on motor recovery of the hemiplegic upper extremity function,' *Australian Occupational Therapy Journal*, 61(2), pp.38–48.

24. Butler, A.J. and Page, S. J. (2006), 'Mental Practice With Motor Imagery: Evidence for Motor Recovery and Cortical Reorganization After Stroke,' *Archives of Physical Medicine and Rehabilitation*, 87(12), pp.2–11.

25. Hamilton, D.R. (2018), *The Five Side Effects of Kindness*, London: Hay House UK and Hamilton, D.R. (2019), *The Little Book of Kindness*, London: Gaia.

26. Morewedge, C.K., et al. (2010), 'Thought for food: imagined consumption reduces actual consumption,' *Science*, 330(6010), pp.1530–1533.

27. Eremin, O., et al. (2009), 'Immuno-modulatory effects of relaxation training and guided imagery in women with locally advanced breast cancer undergoing multimodality therapy: a randomized controlled trial,' *The Breast*, 18(1), pp.17–25.

28. N., Pam M.S., 'AFFIRMATION,' in PsychologyDictionary.org, April 7, 2013, https://psychologydictionary.org/affirmation/ [Accessed May 6, 2021]

29. Steele, C.M. (1988), 'The Psychology of Self-Affirmation: Sustaining the Integrity of the Self,' *Advances in Experimental Social Psychology*, 21, pp.261–302.

30. Cascio, C.N., et al. (2015), 'Self-affirmation activates brain systems associated with self-related processing and reward and is reinforced by future orientation,' *Social Cognitive and Affective Neuroscience*, 11(4), pp.621–629.

31. Cooke, R., et al. (2014), 'Self-Affirmation Promotes Physical Activity,' *Journal of Sport and Exercise Psychology*, 36(2), pp.217–223.

32. Epton, T. and Harris, P.R. (2008), 'Self-affirmation promotes health behavior change,' *Health Psychology*, 27(6), pp.746–752.

33. Critcher, C.R. and Dunning, D. (2014), 'Self-Affirmations Provide a Broader Perspective on Self-Threat,' *Personality and Social Psychology Bulletin*, 41(1), pp.3–18.

Chapter 2: Meditation

1. Berkovich-Ohana, A., et al. (2015), 'Repetitive speech elicits widespread deactivation in the human cortex: the "Mantra" effect?' *Brain and Behavior*, 5(7), pp.1–13.

2. Elder, C. (2014), 'Effect of Transcendental Meditation on Employee Stress, Depression, and Burnout: A Randomized Controlled Study,' *The Permanente Journal*, 18(1), pp.19–23.

3. Bai, Z., et al. (2015), 'Investigating the effect of transcendental meditation on blood pressure: a systematic review and meta-analysis,' *Journal of Human Hypertension*, 29, pp.653–662.

4. Ricard, M., et al. (2014), 'Neuroscience reveals the secrets of meditation's benefits,' *Scientific American*, November, 311(5).

5. ibid.

6. Khoury, B., et al. (2013), 'Mindfulness-based therapy: A comprehensive meta-analysis,' *Clinical Psychology Review*, 33(6), pp.763–771.

7. Goyal, M., et al. (2014), 'Meditation Programs for Psychological Stress and Well-being,' *JAMA Internal Medicine*, 174(3), pp.357–368.

8. Priddy, S.E. (2018), 'Mindfulness meditation in the treatment of substance use disorders and preventing future relapse: neurocognitive mechanisms and clinical implications,' *Substance Abuse and Rehabilitation*, 9, pp.103–114.

9. Hölzel, B.K., et al. (2011), 'Mindfulness practice leads to increases in regional brain gray matter density,' *Psychiatry Research: Neuroimaging*, 191(1), pp.36–43.

10. Garland, E.L., et al. (2020), 'Mind-Body Therapies for Opioid-Treated Pain,' *JAMA Internal Medicine*, 180(1), pp.91–105.

11. Franceschi, C., et al. (2006), 'Inflamm-aging: an Evolutionary Perspective on Immunosenescence,' *Annals of the New York Academy of Sciences*, 908(1), pp.244–254.

12. Creswell, J.D., et al. (2016), 'Alterations in Resting-State Functional Connectivity Link Mindfulness Meditation With Reduced Interleukin-6: A Randomized Controlled Trial,' *Biological Psychiatry*, 80(1), pp.53–61.

13. Dusek, J.A., et al. (2008), 'Genomic counter-stress changes induced by the relaxation response,' *PLoS ONE*, 3(7): e2576.

14. Jacobs, T.L., et al. (2011), 'Intensive meditation training, immune cell telomerase activity, and psychological mediators,' *Psychoneuroendoscrinology*, 36(5), pp.664–681.

15. Le Nguyen, K.D., et al (2019), 'Loving-kindness meditation slows biological aging in novices: Evidence from a 12-week randomized controlled trial,' *Psychoneuroendocrinology*, 108, pp.20–27.

16. Tracey, K.J. (2002), 'The inflammatory reflex,' *Nature*, 420, pp.853–859.

17. De Couck, M., et al. (2018), 'The role of the vagus nerve in cancer prognosis: A systematic and comprehensive review,' *Journal of Oncology*, 2018, pp.1–11.

18. Nestor, J. (2020), *Breath: The New Science of a Lost Art*, New York: Riverhead Books.

19. Kox, M., et al. (2014), 'Voluntary activation of the sympathetic nervous system and attenuation of the innate immune response in humans,' *Proceedings of the National Academy of Sciences*, 111(20), pp.7379–7384.

20. ibid.

Chapter 3: Trapped and Released Emotion

1. Temoshok, L. (1987), 'Personality, coping style, emotion and cancer: towards an integrative model,' *Cancer Surveys*, 6(3), pp.545–567.

2. Kune, G.A., et al. (1991), 'Personality as a risk factor in large bowel cancer: data from the Melbourne Colorectal Cancer Study,' *Psychological Medicine*, 21(1), pp.29–41.

3. Maté, G. (2011), *When the Body Says No: Exploring the Stress-Disease Connection* John Wiley & Sons, Inc., p.126

4. Kneier, W. and Temoshok, L., (1984), 'Repressive coping reactions in patients with malignant melanoma as compared with cardiovascular patients,' *Journal of Psychosomatic Research*, 28(2), pp.145–155.

5. Sahoo, S., et al., (2018), 'Role of personality in cardiovascular diseases: An issue that needs to be focused too!' *Indian Heart Journal*, 70, S471–S477.

6. Keltikangas-jarvinen, L. and Heinonen, K. (2003), 'Childhood Roots of Adulthood Hostility: Family Factors as Predictors of Cognitive and Affective Hostility,' *Child Development*, 74(6), pp.1751–1768.

7. Chida, Y. and Steptoe, A. (2009), 'The association of anger and hostility with future coronary heart disease: A meta analytic review of prospective evidence,' *Journal of the American College of Cardiology*, 53(11), pp.936–946.

8. Smith, T.W., et al. (2006), 'Marital conflict behavior and coronary artery calcification,' Paper presented at the American Psychosomatic Society's 64th annual meeting, Denver, Colorado, March, 2006.

9. 'A Guide to Toxic Stress,' Center on the Developing Child, Harvard University, https://developingchild.harvard.edu/science/key-concepts/toxic-stress/ [Accessed May 3, 2021]

10. Van der Kolk, B. (2014), *The Body Keeps the Score: Mind, brain and body in the transformation of trauma*, London: Penguin, pp.146.

11. Weder, N. et al., (2014), 'Child abuse, depression, and methylation in genes involved with stress, neural plasticity, and brain circuitry,' *Journal of the American Academy of Child & Adolescent Psychiatry*, 53(4), pp.417–424.e5)

12. Felitti, V.J., et al. (1998), 'Relationship of Childhood Abuse and Household Dysfunction to Many of the Leading Causes of Death in Adults,' *American Journal of Preventive Medicine*, 14(4), pp.245–258.

13. Van der Kolk, B. (2014), *The Body Keeps the Score: Mind, brain and body in the transformation of trauma*, London: Penguin, pp.146

14. Dube, S.R., et al. (2009), 'Cumulative Childhood Stress and Autoimmune Diseases in Adults,' *Psychosomatic Medicine*, 71(2), pp.243–250.

15. Burke, N.N., et al., (2016), 'Psychological stress in early life as a predisposing factor for the development of chronic pain: Clinical and preclinical evidence and neurobiological mechanisms,' *Journal of Neuroscience Research*, 95(6), pp.1257–1270.

16. Scott, K.M., et al. (2011), 'Association of childhood adversities and early-onset mental disorders with adult-onset chronic physical conditions,' *Archives of General Psychiatry*, 68, pp.838–844.

17. Nelson III, C.A., et al. (2007), 'Cognitive recovery in socially deprived young children: The Bucharest early intervention project,' *Science*, 318(5858), pp.1937–1940.

18. ibid

19. Pennebaker, J.W. and Evans, J.F. (2014), *Expressive Writing: Words that Heal*, Enumclaw, Idyll Arbor Inc.

20. Pennebaker J.W. and Chung, C.K. (2011), 'Expressive Writing: Connections to Physical and Mental Health,' *The Oxford Handbook of Health Psychology*, Oxford University Press.

21. Church, D., et al. (2018), 'Guidelines for the treatment of PTSD using clinical EFT (Emotional Freedom Techniques), *Healthcare*, 6(4), pp.146–160.

22. Stapleton P., et al. (2021), 'An Initial Investigation of Neural Changes in Overweight Adults with Food Cravings after Emotional Freedom Techniques,' OBM *Integrative and Complementary Medicine*, 4(1), pp.1–14.

Chapter 4: Nature

1. Chan, E.K.F., et al. (2019), 'Human origins in a southern African palaeo-wetland and first migrations,' *Nature*, 575 (7781), pp.185–189.

2. Turner, J., et al. (2015), *Living Psychology: From the Everyday to the Extraordinary*, Milton Keynes: The Open University, p.339.

3. Raanaas, R.K., et al (2012), 'Health benefits of a view of nature through the window: a quasi-experimental study of patients in a residential rehabilitation centre,' *Clinical Rehabilitation*, vol 26, pp.21–32.

4. Grinde, B. and Patil, G. (2009), 'Biophilia: Does Visual Contact with Nature Impact on Health and Well-Being?' *International Journal of Environmental Research and Public Health*, 6(9), pp.2332–2343.

5. Ulrich, R.S. (1984), 'View through a window may influence recovery from surgery,' *Science*, 224 (4647), pp.420–421.

6. Grinde, B. and Patil, G. (2009), 'Biophilia: Does Visual Contact with Nature Impact on Health and Well-Being?' *International Journal of Environmental Research and Public Health*, 6(9), pp.2332–2343.

7. Park, S.H. and Mattson, R.H. (2008), 'Effects of Flowering and Foliage Plants in Hospital Rooms on Patients Recovering from Abdominal Surgery,' *HortTechnology*, 18(4), pp.563–568.

8. Park, S.H., et al. (2004), 'Pain tolerance effects of ornamental plants in a simulated hospital patient room,' *Acta Horticulturae*, 639, pp.241–7.

9. Ulrich, R.S. (1983), 'Aesthetic and affective response to natural environment,' in Altman, I. and Wohlwill, J.F. (eds) *Behaviour and the Natural Environment*, New York: Plenum Publishing, pp.85–126.

10. Thomson Coon, J., et al. (2011), 'Does participating in physical activity in outdoor natural environments have a greater effect on physical and mental well-being than physical activity indoors? A systematic review,' *Environmental Science and Technology*, 45, pp.1761–1772.

11. ibid.

12. Turner, J., et al. (2015), *Living Psychology: From the Everyday to the Extraordinary*, Milton Keynes: The Open University, p.363.

13. Shepley, M., et al. (2019), 'The Impact of Green Space on Violent Crime in Urban Environments: An evidence synthesis,' *International Journal of Environmental Research and Public Health*, 16, pp.5119–5138.

14. Franêk, M., et al. (2018), 'Effect of Traffic Noise and Relaxations Sounds on Pedestrian Walking Speed,' *International Journal of Environmental Research and Public Health*, 15(4), pp.752–764.

15. Saadatmand, V., et al. (2013), 'Effect of nature-based sounds' intervention on agitation, anxiety, and stress in patients under mechanical ventilator support: a randomized controlled trial,' *International Journal of Nursing Studies*, 50, pp.895–904.

16. Farzaneh, M., et al. (2019), 'Comparative Effect of Nature-Based Sounds Intervention and Headphones Intervention on Pain Severity After Cesarean Section: A Prospective Double-Blind Randomized Trial,' *Anesthesiology and Pain Medicine*, 9(2): e67835.

17. Alvarsson, J.J., et al, (2010), 'Stress recovery during exposure to nature sound and environmental noise,' *International Journal of Environmental Research and Public Health*, 7, pp.1036–1046

18. Thoma, M.V., et al. (2013), 'The Effect of Music on the Human Stress Response,' *PLoS ONE*, 8(8): e70156.

19. Bradt, J., et al. (2013), 'Music for stress and anxiety reduction in coronary heart disease patients,' *Cochrane Database of Systematic Reviews*, 12, pp.1–87.

20. Derksen, F., et al. (2013), 'Effectiveness of empathy in general practice: a systematic review,' *British Journal of General Practice*, 63(606), pp.e76–e84.

21. Rakel, D., et al. (2011), 'Perception of empathy in the therapeutic encounter: Effects on the common cold,' *Patient Education and Counseling*, 85(3), pp.390–397.

22. Yang, N., et al. (2018), 'Effects of doctors' empathy abilities on the cellular immunity of patients with advanced prostate cancer treated by orchiectomy: the mediating role of patients' stigma, self-efficacy, and anxiety,' *Patient Preference and Adherence*, 12, pp.1305–1314.

23. Canale, S.D., et al. (2012), 'The Relationship Between Physician Empathy and Disease Complications,' *Academic Medicine*, 87(9), pp.1243–1249.

24. Neumann, M., et al. (2007), 'Determinants and patient-reported long-term outcomes of physician empathy in oncology: A structural equation modeling approach,' *Patient Education and Counseling*, 69(1-3), pp.63–75.

25. Wu, H., et al., (2020), 'Care Is the Doctor's Best Prescription: The Impact of Doctor-Patient Empathy on the Physical and Mental Health of Asthmatic Patients in China,' *Psychology Research and Behavior Management*, 13, pp.141–150.

26. Xu, X., et al., (2020), 'Effects of Patients' Perceptions of Physician–Patient Relational Empathy on an Inflammation Marker in Patients with Crohn's Disease: The Intermediary Roles of Anxiety, Self-Efficacy, and Sleep Quality,' *Psychology Research and Behavior Management*, 13, pp.363–371.

27. Chen, X. et al., (2019) 'Mediating Roles of Anxiety, Self-Efficacy, and Sleep Quality on the Relationship Between Patient-Reported Physician Empathy and Inflammatory Markers in Ulcerative Colitis Patients,' 25, pp.7889–7897.

28. Heid, M. (2017) 'Do Healing Crystals Actually Work?' *TIME*, October 5, 2017.

29. Sharp, D., et al. (2018), 'Complementary medicine use, views, and experiences: a national survey in England,' *BJGP Open*, 2(4), pp.1–19.

30. Dr. Rangan Chatterjee; https://drchatterjee.com

31. Dr. Punam Krishan; https://drpunamkrishan.com

Chapter 5: Reiki

1. Keefe, J. (2017), 'Here are the therapies offered by top hospitals': https://www.statnews.com/2017/03/07/alternative-therapies-chart/ [Accessed April 11, 2021]

2. NHS Royal London Hospital for Integrated Medicine: https://www.uclh.nhs.uk/our-services/our-hospitals/royal-london-hospital-integrated-medicine [Accessed April 11, 2021]

3. American Hospital Association: https://www.aha.org/press-release/2011-09-07-more-hospitals-offering-complementary-and-alternative-medicine-services [Accessed March 11, 2021]

4. Johnson, J.R., et al. (2014), 'The effectiveness of integrative medicine interventions on pain and anxiety in cardiovascular inpatients: a practice-based research evaluation,' *BMC Complementary and Alternative Medicine*, 14(1), pp.486–495.

5. Johnson, J.R., et al. (2014), 'Effects of Integrative Medicine on Pain and Anxiety Among Oncology Inpatients,' *JNCI Monographs*, 2014(50), pp.330–337.

6. Mackay, N., et al. (2004), 'Autonomic Nervous System Changes During Reiki Treatment: A Preliminary Study,' *The Journal of Alternative and Complementary Medicine*, 10(6), pp.1077–1081.

7. Demir Doğan, M. (2018), 'The effect of reiki on pain: A meta-analysis,' *Complementary Therapies in Clinical Practice*, 31, pp.384–387.

8. Billot, M., et al. (2019), 'Reiki therapy for pain, anxiety and quality of life,' *BMJ Supportive & Palliative Care*, 9, pp.434–438.

9. Sagkal Midilli, T. and Ciray Gunduzoglu, N. (2016), 'Effects of Reiki on Pain and Vital Signs When Applied to the Incision Area of the Body After Cesarean Section Surgery,' *Holistic Nursing Practice*, 30(6), pp.368–378.

10. Lacorossi, L., et al. (2017), 'The impact of Reiki on side effects in patients with head-neck neoplasia undergoing radiotherapy: a pilot study,' *Professioni Infermieristiche*, 70(3), pp.214–221.

11. Tsang, K.L., et al. (2007), 'Pilot Crossover Trial of Reiki Versus Rest for Treating Cancer-Related Fatigue,' *Integrative Cancer Therapies*, 6(1), pp.25–35.

12. Olson, K., et al. (2003), 'A phase II trial of reiki for the management of pain in advanced cancer patients,' *Journal of Pain and Symptom Management*, 26(5), pp.990–997.

13. Zucchetti, G., et al. (2019), 'The Power of Reiki: Feasibility and Efficacy of Reducing Pain in Children With Cancer Undergoing Hematopoietic Stem Cell Transplantation,' *Journal of Pediatric Oncology Nursing*, 36(5), pp.361–368.

14. Vergo, M.T., et al. (2018), 'Immediate Symptom Relief After a First Session of Massage Therapy or Reiki in Hospitalized Patients: A 5-Year Clinical Experience from a Rural Academic Medical Center,' *The Journal of Alternative and Complementary Medicine*, 24(8), pp.801–808.

15. Vitale, A.T. and O'Connor, P.C. (2006), 'The effect of Reiki on pain and anxiety in women with abdominal hysterectomies: a quasi-experimental pilot study,' *Holistic Nursing Practice*, 20(6), pp.263–272.

16. Baldwin, A.L., et al. (2017), 'Effects of Reiki on Pain, Anxiety, and Blood Pressure in Patients Undergoing Knee Replacement,' *Holistic Nursing Practice*, 31(2), pp.80–89.

17. Notte, B.B., et al. (2016), 'Reiki's effect on patients with total knee arthroplasty,' *Nursing*, 46(2), pp.17–23.

18. Zins, S., et al. (2018), 'Reiki for Pain During Hemodialysis: A Feasibility and Instrument Evaluation Study,' *Journal of Holistic Nursing*, 37(2), pp.148–162.

19. Jahantiqh, F., et al. (2018), 'Effects of Reiki Versus Physiotherapy on Relieving Lower Back Pain and Improving Activities Daily Living of Patients With Intervertebral Disc Hernia,' *Journal of Evidence-Based Integrative Medicine*, 23, pp.1–5.

20. Richeson, N.E., et al. (2010), 'Effects of Reiki on Anxiety, Depression, Pain, and Physiological Factors in Community-Dwelling Older Adults,' *Research in Gerontological Nursing*, 3(3), pp.187–199.

21. Bremner, M.N., et al. (2016), 'Effects of Reiki With Music Compared to Music Only Among People Living With HIV,' *Journal of the Association of Nurses in AIDS Care*, 27(5), pp.635–647.

22. Gillespie, E.A., et al. (2007), 'Painful Diabetic Neuropathy: Impact of an alternative approach,' *Diabetes Care*, 30(4), pp.999–1001.

23. HeartMath Institute, 'Science of the Heart' https://www.heartmath. org/research/science-of-the-heart/energetic-communication/ [Accessed April 11, 2021]

24. Christakis, N.A. and Fowler, J.H. (2008), 'Dynamic spread of happiness in a large social network: longitudinal analysis over 20 years in the Framingham Heart Study,' *British Medical Journal*, 337, pp.a2338–a2346.

25. McCraty, R. (2003), 'The Energetic Heart: Bioelectromagnetic Interactions Within and Between People,' *The Neuropsychotherapist*, 6(1). pp.22–42

26. Morris, S.M. (2010), 'Achieving collective coherence: Group effects on heart rate variability coherence and heart rhythm synchronization,' *Alternative Therapies in Health and Medicine*, 16(4), pp.62–72.

Chapter 6: Crystals

1. Schwemer, D. (2014), 'Witchcraft in Mesopotamia': https://www.asor. org/anetoday/2014/09/witchcraft-in-ancient-mesopotamia/ [Accessed April 11, 2021]

2. Glencairn Museum (2020), 'Sacred Adornment: Jewelry as Belief in Ancient Egypt': Glencairnmuseum.org. [Accessed April 11, 2021]

3. Online Etymology Dictionary: https://www.etymonline.com/ search?q=crystal [Accessed April 11, 2021]

4. Glick, Thomas F., et al. (2014), *Medieval Science, Technology, and Medicine: An Encyclopedia*. Abingdon: Routledge, p.306.

5. Grant, R.E. (1982), 'Tuuhikya: The Hopi Healer.' *American Indian Quarterly*, 6 (3/4): 293, 301. https://www.jstor.org/stable/1183643 [Accessed April 11, 2021]

6. Thomas, M. (2017), 'Why are Young People So Into Healing Crystals?' https://psmag.com/news/why-are-young-people-so-into-healing-crystals [Accessed April 11, 2021]

7. Wunderman Thompson (2017), 'The Future 100: Trends and Change to Watch in 2017': https://intelligence.wundermanthompson.com/trend-reports/future-100-2017/ [Accessed April 11, 2021]

8. Davies, K. and Freathy, P. (2014), 'Marketplace Spirituality: challenges for the New Age retailer,' *The Service Industries Journal*, 34(15), pp.1185–1198.

9. Woodford, C. (2020), 'Quartz clocks and watches': https://www.explainthatstuff.com/quartzclockwatch.html [Accessed April 11, 2021]

10. Beiser, V. (2018), 'The Ultra-Pure, Super-Secret Sand that Makes Your Phone Possible': https://www.wired.com/story/book-excerpt-science-of-ultra-pure-silicon/ [Accessed April 11, 2021]

11. University of Southampton (2015), 'Research is clear on the study of crystals': ihttps://www.southampton.ac.uk/news/2015/12/crystallography-homepage.page [Accessed April 11, 2021]

12. ibid.

13. Tokyo Institute of Technology (2017), 'Quartz crystals at the Earth's core power its magnetic field': https://phys.org/news/2017-02-quartz-crystals-earth-core-power.html ([Accessed April 11, 2021]

14. Rowe, C.D., et al. (2019), 'Earthquake lubrication and healing explained by amorphous nanosilica,' *Nature Communications*, 10(1), pp.320–330.

15. Maffei, M.E. (2014), 'Magnetic field effects on plant growth, development and evolution,' *Frontiers in Plant Science*, 5, 445.

16. Mridha, N., et al., (2016), 'Pre-sowing static magnetic field treatment for improving water and radiation use efficiency in chickpea (Cicer arietinumL.) under soil moisture stress,' *Bioelectromagnetics*, 37(6), pp.400–408.

17. Magdalena, M., et al. (2016), 'Stimulation with a 130-mT magnetic field improves growth and biochemical parameters in lupin (Lupinus angustifolius L.),' *Turkish Journal of Biology*, 40, pp.699–705.

18. Islam, M., et al. (2020), 'The Geomagnetic Field Is a Contributing Factor for an Efficient Iron Uptake in Arabidopsis thaliana,' *Frontiers in Plant Science*, 11, 325.

19. Freitas, A.M.B., et al. (1999), 'The influence of magnetic field on crystallization from solutions,' Paper presented at the International Conference of Industrial Crystallization, September 1999, England.

20. Wang, C.X., et al. (2019), 'Transduction of the Geomagnetic Field as Evidenced from alpha-Band Activity in the Human Brain,' *eNeuro*, 6(2), pp.1–23.

21. Gilder, S.A., et al. (2018), 'Distribution of magnetic remanence carriers in the human brain,' *Nature Scientific Reports*, 8(1), 11363.

22. Ritz, T., et al. (2009), 'Magnetic Compass of Birds Is Based on a Molecule With Optimal Directional Sensitivity,' *Biophysical Journal*, 96, pp.3451–3457

23. Jorna, R.J. (1987), 'Symbols in the Mind: What are we talking about?' *Current Issues in Theoretical Psychology*, pp.135–150.

24. Hamilton, D.R. (2018), *How Your Mind Can Heal Your Body*, 2nd edition, London: Hay House UK.

25. Shankar, M.U., et al. (2009), 'The influence of color and label information on flavor perception,' *Chemosensory Perception*, 2, pp.53–58

26. DuBose, C., et al. (1980), 'Effects of colorants and flavorants on identification, perceived flavor intensity, and hedonic quality of fruit-flavored beverages and cake,' *Journal Food Science*, 45: pp.1393–1399.

27. Hall, R. (1958), 'Flavor research and food acceptance: A survey of the scope of flavor and associated research, compiled from papers presented in a series of symposia given in 1956–1957.' Reinhold, New York, pp.224–240.

28. Labrecque, L.I. and Milne, G.R. (2012), 'Exciting red and competent blue: The importance of colour in marketing,' *Journal of the Academy of Marketing Science*, 40, pp.711–727.

29. ibid.

30. Grohol, J.M. (2008), 'Can Blue-Colored Light Prevent Suicide?' https://psychcentral.com/blog/can-blue-colored-light-prevent-suicide#1 [Accessed April 11, 2021]

31. Sutter, J.D. (2010), 'Why Facebook is Blue: Six Facts about Mark Zuckerberg': https://edition.cnn.com/2010/TECH/social.media/09/20/zuckerberg.facebook.list/index.html [Accessed April 11, 2021]

32. French, C.C., et al. (2001), 'Hypnotic susceptibility, paranormal beliefs, and reports of "crystal power."' *Proceedings of the British Psychological Society*, 9(2), 186.

33. Kuman, M. (2018), 'Measuring the effects of crystals on the body's electromagnetic field (EMF),' *Journal of Natural and Ayurvedic Medicine*, 2(2), pp.1–4.

Chapter 7: How Perception Shapes Your Reality

1. Ramachandran, V.S. (2012), 'Colored halos around faces and emotion-evoked colors: A new form of synesthesia,' *Neurocase*, 18(4), pp.352–358.

2. Bubl, E., et al. (2010), 'Seeing gray when feeling blue? Depression can be viewed in the eye of the diseased,' *Biological Psychiatry*, 68(2), pp.205–208.

3. Withgott, J. (2000), 'Taking a bird's eye view: Recent studies reveal a surprising new picture of how birds see the world,' *Bioscience*, 50(10), pp.854–859.

4. Evans, R.B. (1990), 'William James, "The Principles of Psychology," and experimental psychology,' *The American Journal of Psychology*, 103(4), pp.433–447.

5. Swanson, A. (2015), 'Why half of the life you experience is over by age 7': https://www.washingtonpost.com/news/wonk/wp/2015/07/23/haunting-images-show-why-time-really-does-seem-to-go-faster-as-you-get-older/ [Accessed April 11, 2021].

6. Hoffman, D. (2019), *The Case Against Reality: How evolution hid the truth from our eyes*. London: Allen Lane.

7. ibid.

Chapter 8: Consciousness

1. Goff, P. (2019), *Galileo's Error: Foundations for a New Science of Consciousness*, London: Rider.

2. Penrose, R. (2020), 'What is Reality?' in *The Essential Guide No.1: 'The Nature of Reality,'* London: New Scientist.

3. ibid.

4. Chalmers, D. (2019), 'Idealism and the mind-body problem,' in Seager, W. (ed), *The Routledge Handbook of Panpsychism*. New York: Routledge, pp.353–373.

5. ibid.

6. Maharaj, N. (Sri) (1999), *I Am That*. Mumbai: Chetana Pvt Ltd.

7. Kastrup, B. (2019), *The Idea of the World*. Alresford: Iff Books.

8. ibid.

9. Maharshi, R. (Sri) (1988), *Be As You Are: the Teaching of Sri Ramana Maharshi*. London: Penguin.

10. Moorjani, A. (2012), *Dying To Be Me*. London: Hay House UK.

11. Tolle, E. (1997), *The Power of Now: A Guide to Spiritual Enlightenment*. Vancouver: Namaste Publishing.

12. His Holiness the Dalai Lama (1999), *Ethics for the New Millennium*. New York: Riverhead Books.

Chapter 9: Telepathy, Distant Healing, and Prayer

1. Duane, T.D. and Behrendt, T. (1965), 'Extrasensory Electroencephalographic Induction between Identical Twins,' *Science*, 150(3694), p.367.

2. Grinberg-Zylberbaum, J. (1982), 'Psychophysiological correlates of communication, gravitation, and unity,' *Psychoenergetics*, 4, pp.227–256.

3. Grinberg-Zylberbaum, J. and Ramos, J. (1987), 'Patterns of Interhemispheric Correlation During Human Communication,' *International Journal of Neuroscience*, 36(1–2), pp.41–53.

4. Smith, J. (2005), 'Telepathy: a new way of seeing': www.theecologist.org/2005/sep/01/telepathy-new-way-seeing [Accessed April 11, 2021]

5. Sheldrake, R. (1999), 'I'm thinking…': www.newscientist.com/article/mg16322015-100-im-thinking/ [Accessed April 11, 2021]

6. Christov-Moore, L., et al. (2014), 'Empathy: Gender effects in brain and behavior,' *Neuroscience & Biobehavioral Reviews*, 46, pp.604–627.

7. Van Der Post, L. (1958), *The Lost World of the Kalahari*. London: Penguin.

8. Sheldrake, R. (2003), The Sense of Being Stared At: And other aspects of the extended mind. London: Arrow Books, pp.103–104. *See also,* Sheldrake, R. and Smart, P. (2003), 'Experimental tests for telephone telepathy, *Journal of the Society for Psychical Research*, 67, pp.184–199 and Sheldrake, R. and Smart, P. (2003), 'Videotaped experiments on telephone telepathy,' *The Journal of Parapsychology*, 67(1), 187–206.

9. Sheldrake, R. (2000), *Dogs That Know When Their Owners Are Coming Home*. London: Arrow Books.

10. Achterberg, J., et al. (2005), 'Evidence for Correlations Between Distant Intentionality and Brain Function in Recipients: A Functional Magnetic Resonance Imaging Analysis,' *The Journal of Alternative and Complementary Medicine*, 11(6), pp.965–971.

11. Grinberg-Zylberbaum, J., et al. (1994), 'The Einstein-Podolsky-Rosen Paradox in the Brain: The transferred potential,' *Physics Essays*, 7(1), pp.422–428.

12. Standish, L.J., et al. (2003), 'Evidence of correlated functional magnetic resonance imaging signals between distant human brains,' *Alternative Therapies*, 9(1), pp.121–125.

13. Christakis, N.A. and Fowler, J.H. (2008), 'Dynamic spread of happiness in a large social network: longitudinal analysis over 20 years in the Framingham Heart Study,' *British Medical Journal*, 337, pp.a2338–a2346, and Rosenquist, J.N. (2010) 'Social network determinants of depression,' *Molecular Psychiatry*, 16(3), pp.273–281.

14. Richards, T.L., et al., (2005), 'Replicable Functional Magnetic Resonance Imaging Evidence of Correlated Brain Signals Between Physically and Sensory Isolated Subjects,' *The Journal of Alternative and Complementary Medicine*, 11(6), pp.955–963.

15. Dossey, L. (1997), 'The Return of Prayer,' *Alternative Therapies in Health and Medicine*, 3(6), pp.10–17, 113–120.

16. Schwarz, B.E. (1967), 'Possible telesomatic reactions,' *Journal of the Medical Society of New Jersey*, 64, pp.600–603.

17. Dossey, L. (1996), 'Notes on the journey: What's love got to do with it?' *Alternative Therapies*, 2(3), pp.8–15.

18. Roberts, L., et al. (2009), 'Intercessory prayer for the alleviation of ill health,' *Cochrane Database of Systematic Reviews*, 2, pp.1–58.

19. Byrd, R.C. (1988), 'Positive therapeutic effects of intercessory prayer in a coronary care unit population,' *Southern Medical Journal*, 81(7), pp.826–829.

20. Krucoff, M.W., et al. (2005), 'Music, imagery, touch and prayer as adjuncts to interventional cardiac care: the monitoring and actualization of noetic trainings (MANTRA) II randomized study,' *The Lancet*, 366, pp.211–217.

21. Benson, H., et al. (2006), 'Study of the therapeutic effects of intercessory prayer (STEP) in cardiac bypass patients: A multicenter randomized trial of uncertainty and certainty of receiving intercessory prayer,' *American Heart Journal*, 151, pp.934–942.

22. Radin, D. (2018), *Real Magic: Ancient Wisdom, Modern Science, and a Guide to the Secret Power of the Universe*. New York: Harmony.

23. Radin, D., et al., (2008), 'Compassionate Intention As a Therapeutic Intervention by Partners of Cancer Patients: Effects of Distant Intention on the Patients' Autonomic Nervous System,' *Explore*, 4(4), pp.235–243.

24. Radin, D. (2018), *Real Magic: Ancient Wisdom, Modern Science, and a Guide to the Secret Power of the Universe*. New York: Harmony.

25. Dunne, B.J. and Jahn, R.G. (2005), 'Consciousness, information, and living systems,' *Cellular and Molecular Biology*, 2005, 51(7), pp.703–714.

26. Jahn, R.G. (1995), 'Report on the Academy of Consciousness Studies,' *Journal of Scientific Exploration*, 9(3), pp.393–403.

27. Nelson, L.A. and Schwartz, G.E. (2006), 'Consciousness and the anomalous organization of random events: The role of absorption,' *Journal of Scientific Exploration*, 20(4), pp.523–544.

28. Freedman, M., et al. (2003), 'Effects of frontal lobe lesions on intentionality and random physical phenomena,' *Journal of Scientific Exploration*, 17(4), pp.651–668.

Chapter 10: The Right Conditions

1. Lamb, E. (2012), '5 sigma, what's that?' https://blogs.scientificamerican.com/observations/five-sigmawhats-that/ [Accessed April 11, 2021]

2. Radin, D. (2018), *Real Magic: Ancient Wisdom, Modern Science, and a Guide to the Secret Power of the Universe*. New York: Harmony, pp.97–100.

3. Utts, J. (2016), 'Appreciating Statistics,' *Journal of the American Statistical Association*, 111(516), pp.1373–1380.

4. *Evening Standard* (2007), 'Is this really proof that man can see into the future?' https://www.standard.co.uk/hp/front/is-this-really-proof-that-man-can-see-into-the-future-6580042.html

5. Schlitz, M.J. and Honorton, C. (1992), 'Ganzfeld psi performance within an artistically gifted population,' *Journal of the American Society for Psychical Research*, 86, pp.83–98.

6. Lawrence, T. (1993), 'Gathering in the sheep and goats: a meta-analysis of forced choice sheep-goat ESP studies, 1947–1993,' Proceedings of the Parapsychological Association 36th Annual Conference, pp.75–86.

7. Schlitz, M., et al. (2006), 'Of two minds: sceptic – proponent collaboration within parapsychology,' *British Journal of Psychology*, 97(3), pp.313–322.

8. Ibison, M. and Jeffers, S. (1998), 'A double-slit diffraction experiment to investigate claims of consciousness-related anomalies,' *Journal of Scientific Exploration*, 12, pp.543–550.

9. Olver, I.N. and Dutney, A. (2012), 'A randomized, blinded study of the impact of intercessory prayer on spiritual well-being in patients with cancer,' *Alternative Therapies in Health and Medicine*, 18(5), pp.18–27.

10. Miranda, T.P.S., et al. (2019), 'Intercessory Prayer on Spiritual Distress, Spiritual Coping, Anxiety, Depression and Salivary Amylase in Breast Cancer Patients During Radiotherapy: Randomized Clinical Trial,' *Journal of Religion and Health*, 59(1), pp.365–380.

Chapter 11: The Law of Attraction

1. Dar-Nimrod, I. and Heine, S.J. (2006), 'Exposure to Scientific Theories Affects Women's Math Performance,' *Science*, 314(5798), pp.435.

2. Keller, A., et al. (2012), 'Does the perception that stress affects health matter? The association with health and mortality,' *Health Psychology*, 31(5), 677–684.

3. Dyer, W. (2012), *Wishes Fulfilled: Mastering the Art of Manifesting*. London: Hay House UK.

4. Nelson, R. (2008), 'What is the Nature of Global Consciousness?' https://noosphere.princeton.edu/science2.html [Accessed April 11, 2021]

5. Jung, C.G. (1985), *Synchronicity: An Acausal Connecting Principle*. Abingdon: Routledge.

6. Burri, M. (2005), 'Der Pauli-Effekt': http://www.ethistory.ethz.ch/besichtigungen/objekte/paulieffekt/ ([Accessed April 11, 2021]

7. Gamow, G. (2003), *Thirty Years that Shook Physics*. New York: Dover Publications, Inc.

Acknowledgments

The idea for this book wasn't my own – it was that of Michelle Pilley, Managing Director and Publisher of Hay House UK. I arranged a meeting with Michelle in the autumn of 2019, before the pandemic began. I wanted to write a book that would be of real value to people and I knew that Michelle would be able to help – she has her finger on the pulse of all things metaphysical, and is very keenly aware of the topics that people want to know about in the mind, body, spirit, personal growth, and holistic health arena.

An author usually arrives at their publisher with an idea for a book and pitches it. I've done that several times, and I liked that it was sort of the other way round this time. At first, the science behind complementary therapies and practices seemed like a big area to write about – there were so many individual subjects I could potentially cover. In the end, there was only space for some of them, but I hope I've chosen those that give a good representation of the general fields of complementary medicine and alternative ideas.

I had some help along the way. A few friends read an early draft of the book, or specific chapters, and offered some kind and helpful feedback, for which I'm extremely grateful: Bryce Redford, Joe

Hayes, Dr. Ann Hutchison, Kyle Gray, Andy Charles, Angela Walker, Mary McManus, Dr. Donna Hoffman, Bonnie MacGregor, Aimee Stewart, Dr. Punam Krishan, Dr. Nilesh Satguru, and Dr. Gemma Newman.

And thanks also to Dr. Robert Holden. As he did on some of my previous books, Robert has a knack of phoning me just at the point where I need to see something more clearly, or to strengthen a conviction, and he played that role perfectly again with this book.

And as always, my partner, Elizabeth, has been a huge support and inspiration – offering insights, feedback, and often a helpfully skeptical point of view that encouraged me to find better ways of explaining some concepts, and being patient about the very long hours I spent working on the text.

All of the staff at Hay House have been so supportive of me through the years. When readers like a book they praise the author, but there are a great many people behind the scenes in a publishing house who bring it to fruition. So I'm grateful to all the people at Hay House who have helped with this and my other titles.

A special thanks to Julie Oughton for putting her 'cunning plan' into action and giving me six additional weeks to work on the book – without that time, it wouldn't be in its current form. And thanks again to Michelle Pilley for offering detailed notes after reading the initial manuscript – these guided much of the revision I made over that six-week period. And a final thanks to my editor, Debra Wolter, for doing a fantastic job on the edit. I think of the role of an editor much like a skilled sculptor who uses fine sandpaper to smooth over the rough edges of a piece before it can be presented to the world.

Index

ABOUT THE AUTHOR

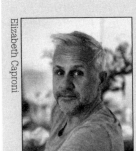

Elizabeth Caproni

David R. Hamilton, Ph.D. was formerly a scientist within the pharmaceutical industry, where he worked at developing drugs for cardiovascular disease and cancer. Inspired by the placebo effect, he left the industry to write books and educate people in how they can harness their mind and emotions to improve their health.

David is now the author of 11 books, including *How Your Mind Can Heal Your Body*, *The Little Book of Kindness*, *The Five Side Effects of Kindness*, and *I Heart Me*. He is the 'Kindness Czar' for *Psychologies* magazine, the 'Life Hacks' columnist for *Soul & Spirit* magazine, and the 'Quantum Science' columnist for *Kindred Spirit* magazine.

He has appeared on Channel 4's *Sunday Brunch* in the UK and CBS *Sunday Morning* in the USA, and is also featured in the documentary *HEAL*.

 DavidRHamiltonPhD

 DavidRHamiltonPhD

 DrDRHamilton

www.drdavidhamilton.com

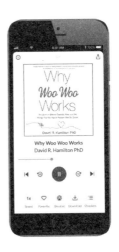

HAY HOUSE

Look within

Join the conversation about latest products,
events, exclusive offers and more.

 Hay House

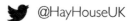 @HayHouseUK

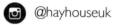 @hayhouseuk

We'd love to hear from you!